Enriched Care Planning for People with Dementia

Bradford Dementia Group Good Practice Guides

Under the editorship of Murna Downs, Chair in Dementia Studies at the University of Bradford, this series constitutes a set of accessible, jargon-free, evidence-based good practice guides for all those involved in the care of people with dementia and their families. The series draws together a range of evidence including the experience of people with dementia and their families, practice wisdom, and research and scholarship to promote quality of life and quality of care.

Bradford Dementia Group offer undergraduate and post graduate degrees in dementia studies and short courses in person-centred care and Dementia Care Mapping, alongside study days in contemporary topics. Information about these can be found on www.bradford.ac.uk/acad/health/dementia.

Enriched Care Planning for People with Dementia

A Good Practice Guide for Delivering Person-Centred Dementia Care

Hazel May, Paul Edwards and Dawn Brooker

Foreword by Murna Downs

Jessica Kingsley Publishers
London and Philadelphia

First published in 2009
by Jessica Kingsley Publishers
116 Pentonville Road
London N1 9JB, UK
and
400 Market Street, Suite 400
Philadelphia, PA 19106, USA

www.jkp.com

Library of Congress Cataloging in Publication Data

May, Hazel.
Enriched care planning : a good practice guide for delivering person-centred care / Hazel May and Paul Edwards.
p. ; cm.
Includes bibliographical references and index.
ISBN 978-1-84310-405-6 (alk. paper)
1. Dementia--Patients--Care. I. Edwards, Paul, R. N. II. Title.
[DNLM: 1. Dementia--Patients--Care. 2. Long-Term Care. 3. Patient-Centered Care. 4. Professional-Patient Relations. WM 220 M466e 2009]
RC521.M388 2009
616.8'3--dc22
2009002561

British Library Cataloguing in Publication Data
A CIP catalogue record for this book is available from the British Library

ISBN 978 1 84310 405 6

Printed and bound in Great Britain by
MPG Books Limited, Cornwall

THIS BOOK IS DEDICATED TO THE MEMORIES OF JAMES FREDERICK YOUNG, VIOLET PEARL EDWARDS AND THOMAS ERNEST EDWARDS: THREE PEOPLE WHO TAUGHT US SO MUCH AND WITHOUT WHOM THIS BOOK WOULD NOT HAVE BEEN WRITTEN.

Contents

List of Templates, Tables and Figures

Templates

Tables and Figures

Acknowledgements

This book has been in progress for at least the last five years and looking back, we feel this was meant to be! If we had completed it, as planned, two years ago it would already by now be out of date. More to the point though, we would not have been in the position to write from a carer's perspective.

The initial work for this book was triggered by a request from two managers of dementia care homes in the Aspects and Milestones Trust in Bristol: Mike Nunn and Lynn Williams. They wanted a complete and integrated training and care-planning 'package' specifically designed to support their staff to deliver high-quality, tailored, person-centred dementia care. Our colleagues from the Bradford Dementia Group, Caroline Baker and Claire Surr worked with us and the nurse managers to design and deliver this, and both the training programme and the care planning templates have developed and improved over time thanks to the thoughtful and detailed feedback and suggestions offered by the Aspects and Milestones staff.

Other colleagues and friends who have supported the writing of this book and contributed to the final version – Fiona Sands, Lorraine Haining, Guy Page and other direct care staff from ExtraCare Charitable Trust, the Royal Hospital Chelsea, Manchester Care and the Royal British Legion.

We would like to thank Errollyn Bruce for supplying ideas on questions that can be used when talking about spiritual needs.

The words of Christine Bryden have been humbling and inspirational and have influenced our work enormously. We thank Christine for this gift.

Very special thanks go to our families Peter, Lauren and Jonathon May and Ruth, Sophie, Beth and Joe Edwards for providing love and support, and for understanding our wish to make a contribution to improving the experience of dementia.

Hazel May, Paul Edwards and Dawn Brooker
Autumn 2008

Foreword

The Department of Health's (2009) National Dementia Strategy emphasises the potential of living well with dementia. There is now a widely recognised need to transform the quality of care and need for an informed and effective workforce. There is an equally pressing need to resource practitioners and professionals with tools to support an emphasis on living well with dementia. *Enriched Care Planning for People with Dementia* is such a tool. Based on Kitwood's person-centred approach, it provides a practical guide to ensuring people live well with dementia.

Enriched Care Planning for People with Dementia provides a concrete and practical framework to work with people with dementia in assessing and addressing the biological, psychological and social aspects of their lives. Having been developed over several years in collaboration with family carers, practitioners and professionals, it is an effective guide to person-centred care planning.

Enriched Care Planning for People with Dementia could not come at a better time with the field poised and determined to make a difference to the well being of people with dementia and their families. I am delighted to welcome you to this book.

Murna Downs
Chair in Dementia Studies,
Bradford University
May 2009

Introduction

Despite important worldwide contributions and developments in the field of dementia care, workers in the field and the public at large remain poorly resourced and supported. This means that many of those who provide care for people with dementia need more awareness, understanding and skills to deliver person-centred care in the years ahead.

Nevertheless, this has been an impressive last fifteen years for professionals in the field; we have seen the evolution of specialised services for people who have dementia and the generalisation of person-centred care as the modern and acceptable response to dementia. We now have a considerable body of evidence suggesting that many people with dementia can tell us about their experiences (Keady 1996; Harris 2002; Sabat 2001) and can report on their own quality of life meaningfully (Mozley *et al.* 1999). This has broadened our perspective as more and more people living with dementia articulate their experience telling of the need to be understood as a 'whole person'; to be with familiar trusted carers; to receive seamless health and social care that is respectful, timely and appropriate and to be allowed to take an active and central role in their own care planning:

> With the stress of many activities at once, I become very focused, trying with all the brain I have left to concentrate. Telling me to rest won't help, but helping me to complete the task will. (Bryden 2005, p.111)

> So I said, 'fine, the health service have done my care plan', he said, 'oh have they, who did that?' So I told him the nurse who had done it and he said 'oh, can you give me her telephone number?' I said 'I'll do better than that, I will get her on the phone and you can talk to her'. So I actually got her on the phone, put the phone in his hand so that he could actually talk to my health worker. (person with dementia) (Alzheimer's Society 2008, p.32)

On the positive side, we have been able to broaden our repertoire, looking to the arts and a variety of psychosocial approaches to enrich practice and a wide range of theoretical frameworks to extend our understanding. There are now a great many national and international publications, conferences and training resources available to support people living with dementia. Somehow though, much of this has failed to filter through to the coalface where the reality within many ordinary care settings, including family homes, is that delivering person-centred care remains an ideal rather than a reality. Bridging the gap between theory and practice has been, and continues to be, a challenge to achieve. As Brooker commented, 'a cursory look around service provision or a discussion with people with dementia and their families suggests that people with dementia are not valued by society' (Brooker 2006, p.31).

Enriched Care Planning for People with Dementia is a resource for those people living with dementia and their carers; it has been found to bridge both the gap between theory and practice and that between health and social care models by providing a practical resource rooted in psychosocial and biomedical theory. In this good practice guide, the key areas of focus for providing person-centred care are described and a process for profiling, identifying and documenting the health, cognitive, social and psychological needs of the person is offered. This, we believe, provides a long-awaited structure for hands-on carers to deliver person-centred care within an inclusive process that enables optimum participation for the person with dementia.

Enriched Care Planning for People with Dementia has been designed and piloted over a five-year period within a range of different dementia care settings including nursing and residential homes; housing schemes and with family carers.

This guide draws from real case examples describing in detail the enriched care planning process and comes with a set of enriched care planning templates to help the person and their carer(s) through the steps of collecting and documenting the information needed for effective person-centred care planning.

A NOTE ON TERMINOLOGY

The term 'carer' is used to refer to any person who is in the role of helping the person who has dementia. This includes professional and paid workers, family carers, friends and advocates.

Chapter 1

What is Enriched Care Planning?

ENRICHED CARE PLANNING – A MEANS TO AN END

Enriched care planning is a means to an end which is delivering person-centred care. Person-centred care is care that values people regardless of age or cognitive ability; is individualised recognising that each individual is unique; includes the perspective of the person with dementia as central to all care planning; values the person as being able to live a life that has meaning and provides a supportive social environment to enable people to experience relationships (Brooker 2006).

This definition of person-centred care describes four essential elements:

1. **Valuing** people with dementia and those who care for them; promoting their citizenship rights and entitlements regardless of age or cognitive impairment or ability.

2. Treating people as **individuals**; appreciating that all people have a unique history and personality, physical and mental health and social and economic resources.

3. Looking at the world from the **perspective** of the person and listening to their 'voice', recognising that each person's experience has its own psychological validity, that people act from their own perspective, and that empathy with the individual's perspective has its own therapeutic potential.

4. Recognising that all human life is grounded in relationships and that people need to live in a **social** environment which both compensates for their impairment and fosters opportunities for personal growth.

A good way to describe and talk about these four elements of person-centred care is to use **VIPS** (Very Important Persons) as a memory jogger because these letters are also the first letters for **V**aluing, **I**ndividuals, **P**erspective and **S**ocial.

PERSON-CENTRED CARE BRINGS WELL-BEING

Well-being is about how a person is faring generally in this current phase of life and means feeling relatively calm, comfortable and at peace. Ill-being means being disengaged and experiencing predominantly negative mood states. Living with dementia does not inevitably result in ill-being; it is more likely that inadequate care delivered in a culture where physical tasks are valued but relationships between the person and their carer(s) are not causes ill-being. (Edvardsson, Winblad and Sandman 2008). In our research and practice development work with the Bradford Dementia Group, we see many people who have dementia experiencing well-being when person-centred care is delivered (Ballard *et al.* 2001; Brooker, Woolley and Lee 2007; Surr 2006).

THE FOCUS FOR PERSON-CENTRED CARERS

Person-centred care is more than being nice or being kind; it requires the whole community of people in which the person with dementia is living to pay special attention to the quality of all relationships, to preserving personhood, promoting inclusion, reducing disability and responding to behaviour on the basis that something important is being communicated.

Relationships

Giving and receiving care is emotional and this applies to the relationships between people who have dementia and those in the role of providing support. How people who have dementia and their carers interact and get along together has a significant effect on the well-being of both parties. The enriched care planning approach takes this seriously and provides a structure for exploring the quality of 'life at the moment' for the person who has dementia.

Preserving personhood

A crucial aspect of being person centred is helping each person to continue to engage with their world so that their sense of self, of personhood and their inner world is kept intact. This means that carers need to find ways of maximising opportunities for engagement so that each individual experiences themselves as being alive and being a person – belonging to the 'personhood club'. This might simply involve maintaining eye contact while helping the person to eat food or knowing the person's life story and using this information to develop a relationship. This degree of individual attention to detail is part of enriched care planning.

Inclusion

In a person-centred care setting, part of the carer's role is to make sure that each individual is brought into the social world rather than just leaving this to chance. This is achieved either verbally with welcomes and invitations to join in through the day or non-verbally by beckoning, holding hands, making eye contact. The goal is to make each person feel that they are accepted as an individual and that they belong in the community.

Contrary to what people might think, people who have dementia can communicate views and feelings about what is happening in their lives (Alzheimer's Society 2008; Barnett 2000; Brod *et al.* 1999; Mozley *et al.* 1999). Person-centred care should be negotiated and agreed openly and in collaboration with the person who has dementia. When using the enriched care planning approach, care staff and/or family members are guided to work in direct partnership with the person who has dementia.

Reducing disability

Disability for the person who has dementia is brought about by the interplay between the person's impairment and their environment. Adaptations to the environment, including the way in which the person is approached and communicated with, can dramatically reduce needless disability caused by a poor care environment. For example, uplift lighting does not cast shadows and for somebody with visual impairment (which is the case for some people who have dementia) this kind of lighting can reduce feelings of fear and distress brought on by being unable to process the sudden appearance of dark shadows. Similarly, when a carer adopts a running commentary which is a simple talking description of what is happening, a person with short-term memory impairment is less likely to feel disorientated and anxious. These are both examples of adaptations that may be appropriate when delivering person-centred care. An Enriched Care Plan will include clear descriptions of adaptations like these that the carer(s) need to make to maximise comfort and promote independence and activity for the person who has dementia.

Believing that all behaviour has meaning

Communication is a fundamental human need and we are all born with a powerful and innate need to connect with the world in which we live. When a person's verbal skills deteriorate their actions can become a vital way of communicating and remaining connected to the world around and many people who have dementia have to rely more on using actions or behaviour to do this. What is so often termed as 'challenging behaviour' in many care settings is more likely to be understood as an expression of physical or emotional discomfort in a person-centred one. Enriched care planning takes account of this, values all behaviour as being meaningful and will produce a support or care plan that seeks to find out more about why a person is behaving in a certain way, or documents clear person-centred and individualised responses to expressions of discomfort such as calling out, weeping, sleeping excessively or repetitive self-stimulation.

ENRICHED CARE PLANNING – A PROCESS

Enriched care planning has been developed as a direct result of using the Enriched Model of Dementia (Kitwood 1997) in dementia care settings around the UK. We have used the model to help workforce teams to move forward from old culture to new culture practice. Old culture practice arises from a one-dimensional view of dementia which pre-judges all that the person says and does as a consequence of having a mind that no longer functions properly. This stance opens the door for all sorts of inappropriate and inadequate approaches and responses that can at best only be described as depersonalising.

The enriched model is a psychosocial model that gives equal importance to the neurological, physiological, psychological and sociological components of human existence. All of these factors have an effect on the experience of dementia. The components of the Enriched Model of Dementia are health, life story, personality, neurological impairment and social psychology which is another way of describing the social and psychological quality of 'life at the moment'. Enriched care planning provides a framework for helping the person who has dementia and their carer(s) to consider each of these in detail as a basis for identifying and meeting current needs.

The Enriched Model of Dementia and its relationship to the Enriched Care Planning Framework is illustrated in Figure 1.1.

Enriched care planning is not just a one-off event, it is a process that takes time and care and it should be ongoing, rather like building a house. If the house is well designed with strong foundations it will be lasting and fit for purpose. Enriched care planning provides a good design and strong foundations for delivering person-centred care.

Enriched care planning involves five stages, as illustrated in Figure 1.2.

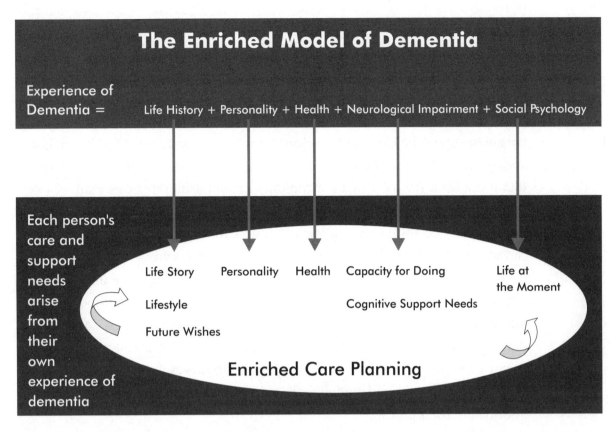

Figure 1.1: The Enriched Model of Dementia and its relationship to the Enriched Care Planning Framework

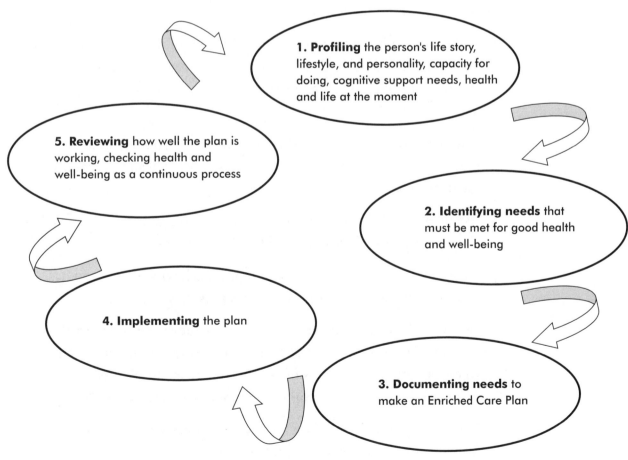

Figure 1.2: The five stages of enriched care planning

ENRICHED CARE PLANNING IS COMMUNICATION

Enriched care planning is more than a paper exercise; writing things down is only part of the process. The final product, the Enriched Care Plan will only be of value if you have communicated directly with the person for whom the care plan has been made. It is important to communicate in a way that you and the person being profiled are both comfortable with and make sure that the quality and quantity of information you collect is 'fit for purpose' in this case meaning that it can form the basis of an uncomplicated and achievable care plan.

The process of profiling can take a long time, and should be ongoing. It is not necessary or always appropriate to set up a formal interview although this can sometimes be helpful if a person is new to the care setting or if their needs have suddenly changed. Even so, this would only be a start; more information can be collected informally during ordinary contact times. Although the information given by the person being profiled needs to be written down, this does not have to happen at the same time; you need to think about how writing things down during a conversation might make the person feel.

Here are some general guidelines to help you when you are trying to gather information for a profile:

- Give the message that you have plenty of time.

- Be prepared to hop around a bit in conversations which are not likely to flow in chronological order.

- Be familiar with the subject matter and layout of the templates so that you don't have to keep flicking through paperwork while you talk; this helps to create a feeling of chatting rather than being 'cross-examined'.

- Have prepared examples of what you are asking about and/or different ways of framing questions ready in your head to accompany the questions.

- Ask questions about people and events that have already been talked about to keep the flow and move the discussion on.

- Take time to recap at intervals and repeat back what the person has said; this often sparks more memories and is very affirming.

- Non-verbal messages are very important to put the person at ease. Lean forward to show interest, smile, nod, make eye contact, laugh where appropriate; give lots of verbal positive feedback – you may be impressed by what the person is telling you – so say so!

- Move on quickly if the information you are asking for seems difficult for the person to know or remember.

Whether or not you make a written record during or after the conversation, it is strongly recommended that you seek consent from the person about making what you have written accessible to that person and anybody else that needs to be involved. It can be helpful to read back what you write to the person and invite comments and suggestions and check that you have correctly represented the information that has been offered. If the person being profiled cannot speak for themselves, the same principles will apply as you communicate through eye contact, touch and sound and seek information from advocates and other carers.

You can use your own forms or you can use some or all of the enriched care planning templates provided with this good practice guide to steer you through this process. These templates are there to help you to piece together a detailed profile from which you can identify needs from which to draw up your plan of action or your final Enriched Care Plan.

There are seven profiling templates and three working templates, plus an Enriched Profile and Care Plan Cover Sheet that is also provided as a pull-out. Use this as a front sheet for each individual's Enriched Care Plan. The profiling templates lay out all the questions you may need to ask and issues you may need to consider during the first step of profiling the person.

Use the working templates to document what the person wants other people to know on a day-to-day basis and what their carers need to do to provide person-centred care. These templates should be owned by and accessible to the person. All of the templates can be found as pull-outs for photocopying at the back of this good practice guide.

Profiling templates

- Life Story Profile
- Lifestyle and Future Wishes Profile
- Personality Profile
- Health Profile
- Capacity for Doing Profile
- Cognitive Ability Profile
- Life at the Moment Profile

Working templates

- Enriched Profile and Care Plan Cover Sheet
- Brief Profile Sheet

- Key Information Sheet

- The Enriched Care Plan

The next chapters deal in detail with the whole process of profiling, identifying needs, and documenting actions in relation to life story, lifestyle and future wishes, personality, health, capacity for doing, cognitive ability and life at the moment. We will look at the information you need to gather and why it is important to do so as well as providing instruction and guidance for using each of the seven profiling templates.

The final chapter includes discussion points and guidance for implementing and reviewing the plan both of which are important parts of the enriched care planning process.

SUMMARY

- Enriched care planning is a process for delivering person-centred care.

- The aim is to promote and maintain well-being for the person living with dementia.

- How the carer views dementia and communicates with the person is central to the enriched care planning process.

- The process of enriched care planning is drawn from Kitwood's Enriched Model of Dementia.

- Life story, lifestyle and future wishes, personality, health, capacity for doing, cognitive ability and life at the moment are all key issues in enriched care planning.

- Enriched care planning involves five steps: profiling the person; identifying needs; documenting needs; implementing the plan; reviewing the plan.

- This good practice guide provides profiling templates and working templates to help you work through the enriched care planning process. You can use them as they are, adapt them or combine them with your own documentation.

Chapter 2

Life Story

We each have our own life story – the important experiences and events that have left their mark. Taking time and care to discover the person through life story over time is a non-negotiable part of enriched care planning.

There are two reasons for this. First, drawing from life story is often the most accessible way for a person who has memory problems to communicate and 'be themselves'. The most common types of dementia usually make it hard for the person to file, store and save recent information and events. This leads to short-term memories being lost. It then becomes easy for others to make the mistake of assuming that the person can't remember anything. This isn't true; it is very likely that, given the opportunity the person can and will be able to access older memories and these can reveal so much about who they are. The second reason is because life story can often shed light on situations helping others to understand why a person is behaving or reacting to current events in the way they are.

There has been so much very good material about life story work and a number of excellent life story products published which are highly recommended. You can have a look at these and develop your own way of approaching life story work; you may also have your own ideas and techniques for finding out about and documenting life story material; you can also use the Life Story Profiling Template or perhaps even a combination of all or some of these. What is important is that you do not overlook life story work or leave it for another time or for somebody else to do. Life story work is at the very core of delivering person-centred care and if you take time and care to attend to this seriously and professionally the rewards for you and for the people you care for will be very worthwhile.

The process of building up an individual life story profile can take time and requires skill and insight. In a sense, you are taking on a job that many families share through time: the job of sifting, storing, sharing and retelling important stories within the family group. Sifting what is significant from what isn't should be done from the perspective of the person who has dementia. For example, the names of all the grandchildren and their birthdays may be 'easy' information to find and record but, how important are these names to the person who has dementia? Stories from their own childhood and teenage years and earlier on in their own life that have been rehearsed many times may be far more significant and useful for nurturing the person's sense of identity and well-being. Time and skill are both required for accessing these memories with and for the person who has dementia. Memories are the stuff of our hearts as much as of our minds and people have plenty in their hearts.

Reminiscing is a good way to find out about life story. It is something we all do as part of being human. You can reminisce on a one-to-one basis or in a group activity using it to gently invite responses that may hold clues for significant memories. Reminiscence connects with the essence of the person, focusing on retained memories and social skills. The idea is to keep communication going and to celebrate people's lives as a whole. Objects, sounds, pictures and activities that stimulate all the senses can be used to trigger memories and facilitate communication.

Collecting photos and mementos from current living experiences can build up a sense of identity just as much as and maybe more so than old ones. Also, there may be particular objects in the care setting that the person becomes attached to or shows an interest in; these are all important things to document in the person's life story profile.

When you are talking about life story, it can be a good idea to stop every so often and summarise, feedback and check out what you have heard with the person. This applies whether you are in a one-to-one, group, formal or informal situation and will do much to affirm, acknowledge and support the person.

Life story work ought to be given as much value and priority as physical care and should be an ongoing process. Responding to somebody who is distressed because they cannot find a loved one and does not remember that the loved one has died requires a person-centred approach. You may struggle to provide this if you don't know enough about that particular person. It is tempting to use tactics that quickly take the person out of their distress: 'He'll be here soon' or 'She's just popped out'. It is unhelpful to be blunt and insensitive 'She died three years ago, don't you remember?'

A family member or care worker who knows the person's life story will be able to say 'I remember you telling me about your husband, he worked in the mines didn't he?' This may lead to a dialogue in which the care worker can move on from distant memories to more recent ones; and then to move on to find out what the person wants, what is bothering them; to give emotional support and to gently reorientate the person to where they are now and to what is happening next.

If you are unable to find out about the person's life history, start to build up a profile now. What you find out today will be history tomorrow and may provide important building blocks for helping the person to develop new relationships and establish a sense of identity. One unique idea we have tried is the 'shoe box' approach to life story profiling. This is where an empty box is put out on the unit and staff are asked to jot down small bits of information they discover about the person during their everyday interactions. Once quickly jotted down the bits of paper are put into the box. At the end of a fortnight, all the information can be shared with the person and, with permission, included in the Life Story Template.

Age Exchange is an excellent organisation that offers a range of reminiscence publications and courses. Contact details are included in the list of useful resources at the back of this book.

USING THE LIFE STORY PROFILING TEMPLATE

The Life Story Template has four sections:

- Early Years

- Middle Years

- After Retirement

- Now

In our experience of doing life story work, it is often easier to start off a discussion by focusing on very early memories such as names of grandparents, parents and brothers and sisters than to remember more recent facts and information such as names and ages of grandchildren. So try starting with the very earliest childhood memories bearing in mind that a full scale 'interview' is not necessarily the easiest or most fruitful approach. Life story details can be collected and built up over time – rather like piecing together a big jigsaw with many pieces.

Each of these Life Story Template sections has several themes to help you structure your communication with the person. Bear in mind though that these headings are only there as a guide. Other topics may well come up such as details about significant losses or about how the person has reacted in other situations and coped with change in the past. These also need to be included in the profile and there is a 'Stories' box at the bottom of each section for writing down this kind of information.

You may need to be proactive in contacting family, friends and anybody previously or currently involved in the person's life. Remember that it is good practice to ask for consent from the person to ask others and to write down information about their life.

Here are some guidelines for completing each section.

Early Years

For most people, early days are memorable and significant and give such a good insight into the essence of the person. Talking about immediate family, school friends, journeys to school, teachers, loved and less-loved subjects can be a very fruitful and rewarding experience for both the person talking and the person listening. It may be easier for the person being profiled to access memories about their talents and interests, friends, achievements and aspirations and how they spent their free time and holidays in the context of a general conversation about school days than being asked 'cold'.

Names of grandparents, parents and siblings may come easily, but, if not, you should quickly move on to try and access visual memories such as the house the person lived in. What did it look like? Where did they sleep? What do they remember about the kitchen? Ask questions such as 'What sticks in your mind especially about those days?' 'What were Christmases like?' and so on.

Another route into memory is through emotion and so questions could be asked such as:

- 'Was your father strict?'

- 'Did you and your sister ever get into trouble?'

- 'Did you have a special toy that you really loved?'

- 'Who was your favourite teacher?'

- 'What were you best at in school?'

- 'Do you remember any special friends?'

- 'What did you dream of being when you grew up?'

These questions may evoke particular memories or events from school days such as winning a race, getting into trouble, favourite and dreaded teachers or even wartime experiences. This is the kind of thing you would write in the 'Stories' box.

Here is an example of how you might fill in the Early Years section of the Life Story Template.

Memories of Family and Friends

My Grandparents

James' grandparents lived in Ireland, he never met them, can't remember names. They had a farm, Grandfather went to war, and Grandmother looked after children on the farm.

My Parents

Mother 'Agnes' was soft and gentle but father 'Bert' was very strict, drank and often gave the kids a 'clip'. He was a builder, often disappeared for months at a time. Agnes worked from home sewing for Selfridges. Family home was in Bayswater, London. The house was in Talbot Road, hence referred to as 'Talbot'.

My Brothers and Sisters

James was the oldest of five children. Next came Eileen, then Josie, Malvie, Steven. All quite close in age, tended to stick together with James at the helm.

Other People

Large family so cousins and aunts and uncles were important. James had a special relationship from early on and right through his life with his older cousin Liam and Liam's parents, Aunty Tillie and Uncle John.

Memories of Schooling and Education

My Talents and Interests

James' best subjects were football and art.

My Friends and Teachers

Special friends at junior school were Jack and Eddie, all went to local Catholic junior school half mile away.

My Achievements and Dreams

James was proud to win the Junior Art competition aged seven, he did a pencil picture of Mickey Mouse. He says he dreamed of earning his own money!

Early Years Stories

James' mum told him the story of her childhood living on the farm in Ireland, she looked after eggs sometimes, smuggled them up her jumper and took them to bed to try and hatch them.

Earliest memory of his mum is being chased by her, up the garden path for being naughty. He remembers she was wielding a hairbrush! James often got into trouble with younger sister Josie; they got caught stealing apples from a local farmer's garden.

Middle Years

For some people, memories from middle years can be more difficult to access. Prompts about weddings and births, jobs and particular hobbies will be helpful. Dates and names are less important than descriptions about events and people. So rather than 'When did you get married?' questions like 'Was it a sunny day?' might be easier to handle.

Here are some questions that you might like to use:

- 'Was it sunny that day?'

- 'What did you wear?'

- 'Was the food good?'

- 'Did your best friend come to your wedding?'

Questions about work and leisure can similarly be focused on events and people.

- 'Do you remember your first day at work?'

- 'How did you travel to work?'

- 'What was the colour/make of your first car?'

- 'Tell me about bath time with your children.'

- 'What was your boss like?'

- 'Did you have any time for yourself?'

- 'What did you do to relax?'

- 'What was your best/worst holiday with the children?'

These questions may evoke particular memories or events from this period of time which you would write in the 'Stories' box.

There is a prompt in this section for talking about difficult times and sad days and this kind of conversation really needs to be led by the person you are profiling. Be prepared for memories of sad times to come to the surface and view this as positive. The person must feel safe with you and it is a sign of well-being to be able to experience and show a range of different emotions. Stay with the feeling and then move on, or steer the person to a more neutral or positive memory when it feels comfortable to do so.

Here is an example of how you might fill in the Middle Years section of the Life Story Template.

Memories of Family and Friends

Weddings, Births and Other Special Days

Yvette married in the pouring rain but she says it didn't matter, the cake was the best, made by her sisters Lucy and Margaret, it was cream and white, three layers. Not many people outside the family came to the wedding – couldn't afford it. She remembers the first birth in the family; her sister had a baby girl called Nicola who caused great excitement – Nicola was the apple of everybody's eye. Yvette followed quite soon with her own two children Lizzie and Jason, eighteen months apart.

Difficult Times and Sad Days

Bringing Lizzie and Jason up in the first few years was the most difficult time of her life – Jason never slept. Yvette had moved from the city to the country, given up her job and her husband was a workaholic and not around very much.

Yvette's husband John died young, he was only forty and the children aged seven and nine. He died suddenly at work from a heart attack and Yvette still cries when she remembers this. It has made her anxious about losing people she loves.

Memories of Things I Did

My Work

Yvette's first job was in a shoe shop. She stayed for a while then stopped working to be a mum.

My Hobbies and Holidays

Yvette loved to sing and she played guitar and mandolin which she learned to do by ear. She would love to have family parties at her house and invite everybody, grown-ups and children to sing and play at the parties.

The family would go to Brighton for a week every summer for their holidays. These were all great holidays.

Middle Years Stories

Yvette remembers when Lizzie was born, it was a difficult birth but Lizzie was just beautiful and she couldn't stop looking at her. Her husband John came and picked her up in an old van with Wellington boots on the front seat and they had a row about this. John's mum Di cooked a lovely meal for them all on her first night back home, lamb chops and broccoli and even now this is her favourite comfort food.

Worst holiday was when Yvette and the family went to Margate one year instead of Brighton – Jason was ill with food poisoning and it rained for the whole week.

After Retirement

This is an important life stage sometimes bringing new freedoms to travel, enjoy hobbies, family and such like. The post-retirement years however may also encompass the life stage in which the person you are profiling has started to develop dementia and lost friends and/or close family members. People often have to adapt to further changes at this stage of life such as moving to a smaller house or into a care home and although it is to be hoped that these experiences are positive, they may cause distress.

If the person struggles to access memories from this period, ask them for permission to find out more from others. If consent is given, find out what you can and then share it with the person at an appropriate time. This will equip you to gently continue or finish the story with the person and to support them emotionally if the need arises.

Here are some questions you can ask that may help memories to surface about this stage of life:

- 'Did you work right up until you were sixty/sixty-five years of age?'

- 'When you left the job, did you have a party?'

- 'Did your work mates give you a gift, a clock or something like that?'

- 'Was it nice to stop working, or did you miss it?'

- 'Did you stay living in the same house or did you move?'

- 'What was the best thing you did after you retired?'
- 'Did you get any rest, or were you kept busy with looking after grandchildren?'

If you ask these questions on behalf of the person being profiled you should get consent. Also, consider carefully and discuss together who is the best person to talk to about this life stage. Often, grown-up children are asked but they have a very different perspective!

Here is an example of how you might fill in the After Retirement section of the Life Story Template.

Memories of Family and Friends
Weddings, Births and Other Special Days

James remembers his daughter's wedding and how proud he felt giving her away and making everybody laugh with his witty speech.

His marriage to his second wife Fran also sticks in his mind. They had a quiet registry office wedding then drinks and nibbles back at home in the garden on a lovely summer's day. He felt very happy and excited about moving to Florida with Fran.

He remembers lots of happy days and memories when his daughters and his grandchildren came to visit him in Florida, he made sure they all had a trip to Disney World.

Difficult Times and Sad Days

The end of James' working life as an insurance broker was difficult. He can't remember exactly what happened but he left suddenly and on a bad note.

When James' mum Agnes died he took a long time to get over it. It was especially sad because he was in Florida and he couldn't get back to be with her or go to her funeral.

Memories of Things I Enjoyed
Work, Hobbies and Travel

James finished working as an insurance broker but then spent a lot of time playing golf, planning trips home to the UK and making music and chat tapes to send home to his children. He took up art again and did a special painting for each of his grandchildren.

Special Places and Special Things

James loved visiting his sister Josie in her home in London and this home 'Main Road' became special to him. His other sister Eileen did an oil painting of his early family home, Talbot Road, and this picture too was and still is very special. It brings back happy memories which he likes to talk about.

After Retirement Stories

Josie and her husband Andy and James went to France for a day trip and Andy bought a load of bulbs for his garden. But, when he brought them home, they were onions.

James remembers going to the shoe shop with one of his granddaughters to buy her her first pair of shoes – they were white with a buckle at the side.

Football was still a big thing and James remembers taking his nephews to see Chelsea vs Queens Park Rangers on Boxing Day one year when he was over on a visit from Florida – great day out. Needless to say Chelsea won, Queens Park Rangers was James' team.

Now

These years can be times of change and loss and perhaps the onset of illness or impairment. The focus here should be on trying to access material which is important now. So, it may be more relevant for the person being profiled to be helped to talk about people who they think about. These might be people who are still alive or people who have died. Places may also be important and these might be geographical, such as countries, towns, cities, or particular spaces such as a particular kitchen or garden or bedroom. There may also be activities that the person thinks about, enjoyable and otherwise. Enjoyable activities might include gardening, pottering at home, being with special family or friends. It is not uncommon for some people to be preoccupied with an activity that they can't do or feel they ought to be doing such as collecting children from school, going home, going to bed.

The important thing in this part of the profile is to try to understand what has been happening more recently in their mind, from their perspective.

There are no example questions provided for this section of the Life Story Template. This is because you are part of what is happening now. You shouldn't need to ask questions as such. It is more likely that what is important for the person now will be made explicit through actions and words that you share and observe in your day-to-day caring role.

You should use the 'Stories' section to write down current stories that have meaning for the person.

Here is an example of how you might fill in the Now section of the Life Story Template.

Who and What I Think About

For the past few weeks, James has wanted to talk about his mum and the house where he grew up, Talbot Road. He spends time waiting for his daughters to visit and talking about their jobs, their husbands and their children.

Proudest Achievements

James often talks with pride of how he progressed from age fourteen with no qualifications to being a director of a big city insurance company. He was proud to be able to buy his own house and afford his own car.

Regrets

Falling out with his dad and not properly patching things up before his dad died.

Best Day

Family picnic at Greenwich Park.

Happiest Memories

Growing up in Talbot Road. Playing golf with Cousin Liam.

Recent Stories

James had a great birthday party with his family in July. He especially loved watching his great-grandchildren playing in the garden. He has photographs in his room.

Last week James took part in a quiz and surprised everybody with his knowledge of football. He won the quiz and everybody clapped.

IDENTIFYING AND DOCUMENTING NEEDS FROM THE LIFE STORY PROFILE

When you have finished profiling the person's life story you will need to review this together and then identify together any needs arising that are relevant to the care situation at the moment.

Needs are those things which make or break the day for an individual. It can be helpful to think about yourself here. If you had to rely on others for your health and well-being, what life story issues would be important to you? For most of us, it would be important for people to know about our families, about important achievements and losses and what we are good at. There may be particular events that happened in the past that have a direct bearing on the here and now.

A colleague of ours told a true story about a man called Dennis she once worked with. Dennis was being looked after in an acute hospital setting recovering from a physical illness. She had been asked to help the care team to 'manage' his challenging behaviour. The behaviour was that he was resistive to staff when they tried to get him out of bed in the morning. My colleague worked through the Enriched Model with Dennis and his family and the care team. Eventually, an important piece of information relating to life story came to light. As a young boy, one of Dennis' uncles had thrown him into a swimming pool in an attempt to teach him how to swim. Dennis did not learn to swim; he was traumatised by the incident because he nearly drowned and he spent the rest of his life harbouring a fear of water. This event was affecting how he behaved in the hospital because the floor in his room was blue shiny lino. Dennis was frightened when the staff tried to pull him from his bed because he thought he was going to end up in the water (the blue shiny floor).

Identifying needs

Identifying needs in relation to life story involves linking important events and people from the past with the current situation.

Look back over the life story examples for James and Yvette above and try to identify anything that would be important now.

You should include anything that you need to know more about – perhaps a period of time that the person cannot tell you about. For example, there is very little known about James' marriage to his first wife. If this is something that James says he would like to talk about, and you need more information to help him remember and talk, you should identify this as a need.

Other needs to identify will come from individualised information from the profile.

For James this information might include:

- family orientated

- picture of Talbot Road important

- likes drawing

- interested in and knowledgeable about football, supports Queens Park Rangers

- lived for twenty-five years in Florida.

For Yvette:

- enjoys singing, used to play guitar and mandolin

- favourite comfort food is lamb chops and broccoli

- Brighton is a place that brings happy memories

- worked in a shoe shop before having children.

Relevance for the here and now might be for James' well-being:

- family orientated – comfortable with people around him

- picture of Talbot Road – needs to be able to see this picture in his room

- likes drawing – might like art-type activities and trips

- interested in and knowledgeable about football, supports Queens Park Rangers – will enjoy conversations, activities, pictures involving football especially Queens Park Rangers

- lived for twenty-five years in Florida – will relate to conversations, pictures, news items about Florida.

For Yvette's well-being:

- enjoys singing, used to play guitar and mandolin – will enjoy musical activities, singing, anything to do with guitar or mandolin

- favourite comfort food is lamb chops and broccoli – Yvette will enjoy this as a special meal, and remembering the birth of her first child

- Brighton is a place that brings happy memories – pictures, films, discussions about Brighton will promote Yvette's well-being

- worked in a shoe shop before having children – reminding Yvette about her job in a shoe shop will promote her sense of identity and self-esteem.

Documenting needs

Having identified what is important to the person, you will now need to reflect this in what you write in the three working templates:

- Brief Profile Sheet
- Key Information Sheet
- The Enriched Care Plan.

The Enriched Care Plan Cover Sheet is also provided as a pull-out. Use this as a front sheet for each individual's Enriched Care Plan.

Brief Profile Sheet

There is a space at the top of the Brief Profile Sheet 'Important Issues Relating to my Life Story'. There is only room to briefly summarise the very important things, and you will need to talk to the person and/or their family to decide what these are. For James, it might be 'Grew up in London, large Irish Catholic family in a house called Talbot Road, keeps picture in his room. Important people are mother Tillie, sisters Eileen, Josie and Malvie, brother Steven and cousin Liam. James excelled at art and football as a lad, supported Queens Park Rangers. Spent last twenty-five years living in Florida with second wife Fran.'

Key Information Sheet

There may be people who have come up during profiling of life story that the person may want you to contact, regularly or in emergencies on their behalf. This section is entitled 'People that I may wish to contact'.

For James and Yvette these would be likely to be their siblings and their children.

The other section of relevance in the Key Information Sheet is further down the page and entitled 'Important information that I want people involved in my care to know about'. Again, if anything has come up during profiling of life story that the person feels is very important for others to know about, it can be recorded here. In the example of Dennis and his childhood experience of drowning, his fear of water would have been relevant information for this section.

The Enriched Care Plan

The end product, the Enriched Care Plan, will be drawn from all the profiling that you do in relation to life story, lifestyle and future wishes, personality, health, capacity for doing, cognitive ability and life at the moment. There are just three columns in the plan. On the left hand side is the column entitled 'I need'. The middle column is headed 'My carers will'. The right hand column is for recording a date for review.

At this stage in the enriched care planning process, you only need write in the 'I need' column in relation to needs arising from life story. As already said, these needs will be things that make or break the person's day: things that are important *to* the person. For James, in the 'I need' column, you might write: 'To see my picture of Talbot Road every day.' For Yvette, you might write: 'To have lamb chops and broccoli for dinner sometimes, especially if I am tired or upset.'

SUMMARY

- Drawing from life story is often the most accessible way for a person who has memory problems to communicate and 'be themselves'.

- Life story can often shed light on situations helping others to understand why a person is behaving or reacting to current events in the way they are.

- Life story work ought to be given as much value and priority as physical care and should be an ongoing process.

- It is often easier to access early childhood memories than it is to remember more recent things.

- The life story profiling process provides a framework for accessing important information about Early Years, Middle Years, After Retirement, and Now.

- Identifying needs in relation to life story involves linking important events and people from the past with the current situation.

- The Enriched Care Plan will identify needs arising from life story that are relevant to the care situation at the moment.

Chapter 3

Lifestyle and Future Wishes

A lifestyle is the way in which a person lives, usually affected by the wider cultural context but flavoured with individual practices and preferences that are deeply rooted because they have developed over the duration of the person's lifetime. The focus here is on finding out the detail of what is relevant, important and comfortable currently to the individual. This information needs to be held and known by the immediate carer(s) and forms an important cornerstone of person-centred care. This is especially the case in formal care settings where the cultural undercurrents of day-to-day living may not be familiar or comfortable in the way they automatically are within a family.

The meaning of 'culture' comes from the Latin word 'cultura' which means 'to cultivate'. When we talk about culture, we mean patterns of human activity or a way of life that includes codes of manners, dress, language, religion, rituals, norms of behavior such as law and morality, and systems of belief as well as the arts. If the individual's cultural essence is not understood and respected, the likelihood of behaviour being judged as challenging or inappropriate raises its head again. Cultures are very different for example between eastern and western parts of the world but they can also be different between families living in the same street. For one family, it may be perfectly 'normal' to leave the door open or unlocked when visiting the toilet while, for another, this might be unacceptable, abhorrent even. Individuals coming from such different backgrounds will have very different reactions living in a group situation where it sometimes happens that toilet doors are left unlocked or open when somebody is using the toilet.

Two very important aspects of profiling lifestyle and future wishes, in particular for people who have dementia, are included here and they are **attachment** and **spirituality**. Discussion about patterns of activity relating to attachment and spirituality can lead on quite comfortably and naturally to talking about future wishes which are bound to be closely linked to the person's current lifestyle and to what is culturally acceptable for them. Knowing about these will become very important should the person become less able to communicate their wishes verbally or through action at any time in the future.

These days, it is becoming increasingly important for people to make a Living Will and/or an Advance Directive and to make provision for Lasting Power of Attorney. These are matters which need to be attended to while the person has full mental capacity. As part of the enriched care planning process, it may be appropriate for you to help the person you are profiling to think about and document their future wishes. The Office of the Public Guardian and the Court of Protection, Mind and Age Concern offer advice and information about these matters and their contact details are included in the list of useful resources at the back of this book.

USING THE LIFESTYLE AND FUTURE WISHES PROFILING TEMPLATE

Lifestyle

The first page of the template is for recording information about what is important for the person regarding:

- food and drink
- clothes
- daily living activities
- work-like activities
- relaxing and social activities
- personal attachment figures or objects
- spirituality.

Food and drinks that I like

Include here information about the types of food and drink that the person likes as well as preferred habits and routines. For example it may be that the person does not normally eat breakfast but that they enjoy a biscuit and a cup of coffee at 9.30 am. Or it could be that the person prefers to eat their main cooked meal at 5.00 pm followed by a light supper at 10.00 pm. There may be types of food that the person does not eat for medical, moral or cultural reasons and these should be included in this section. Food or drink used for comfort or 'treats' is important information too. For example, a glass of sherry at 6.00 pm, special cooked dinners on a Sunday or a warm drink of milk and honey on sleepless nights. In this section, you might also include preferences about where and how food is eaten. For example, whether the person wishes to eat alone or in a group, or to eat from a table or from their lap. How the person demonstrates dislike for food may also be relevant. In some cultures it is perfectly acceptable to voice dislike of food while, in others, this is not done – the food is simply left uneaten. Using cutlery may be common practice in some cultures while, in others, using the fingers to eat is the norm.

Clothes I like to wear

Having control over what we wear and being free to dress in a way that confirms who we are is something that most of us take for granted. So, to be living in a world where other people take control of what we wear must feel like a loss of identity. This part of the Lifestyle and Future Wishes Template is there to prompt the carer(s) to find out specifically about the clothes that the person wishes to wear. This should include under and outer garments as well as details of how the person chooses to dress for different occasions and circumstances. This might not be the same as how the person is currently 'being dressed'! Information about how the person dressed in the past may also be useful and relevant. Favourite colours and favourite garments, including footwear, should also be recorded in this section.

My routines for daily living activities

In this section, information about the manner in which the person attends to their personal care should be recorded. Personal care includes activities such as washing, bathing, showering, going to the toilet, dressing, washing/combing/ brushing hair, looking after teeth, applying makeup and shaving. Personal preferences such as 'prefers a bath to a shower' or 'likes to get dressed after breakfast' or 'likes to leave the door open when using the toilet' should be recorded here.[1]

Work-like activities that I need to do routinely

Work-like activities include dusting, sweeping, tidying up, sorting, collecting, storing, checking, watching, fixing, locking up, turning out lights and many more. Our extensive observations of people who have dementia in residential care settings tell us that work-like activities occur frequently and, if supported and encouraged by care staff, that they contribute significantly to well-being.

---

1   Please note information relating to diet, fluid intake, moving around, using the toilet, sleeping, eye sight, hearing, feet, teeth/oral care and skin is included in the Health section.

We refer to them as 'work-like' activities because they are often performed in an industrious and skilled manner, even if the real or actual objects or tools for the job are not available in the care setting. Often, these activities seem to stem from previous occupations. An ex-plumber may spend time checking taps and bath fittings while an ex-lighthouse man may get up at night to check the position of the lights outside the window of the home; one lady may have a strong drive to look after other people or fret about children while another may want to spend time in the office, the kitchen or the laundry. In many old culture care settings, activities such as these have been judged as meaningless or disruptive and actively discouraged. So, it may be important to find out about and record previous work roles such as 'headmaster', 'homemaker' or 'shop worker' as well as any productive or work-like activities that the person currently engages in. These can be activities that the person initiates on their own such as washing up or making the bed, or those that are prompted or random such as 'enjoys helping to lay the table when invited' or 'likes to stack chairs in the dining room during the day'.

Person-centred care means supporting these activities and seeing them as opportunities to strengthen relationships and validate feelings. An Enriched Care Plan will outline clearly ways in which the person's carer(s) can do this.

How I relax

Past and current leisure and social activities that the person has actually taken part in should be included here. These are activities that the person naturally elects to do when not involved in the structured and routine activities of daily living. Although past hobbies would fall into this category, these may not be important to or yearned for by the person at the current time. For example, the person may have enjoyed dancing in the past and now, due to poor mobility, may no longer partake in dancing activities.

However, hobbies that the person cannot engage in anymore should still be included because they provide useful information for activity planning – it could be in this example that the person could be helped to watch TV programmes about ballroom dancing, or to talk about it. So, lifelong leisure pursuits like this, *in addition to current* leisure and social pursuits that the person reports or has been observed to enjoy, such as talking, singing or being with the family, should also be included in this section.

People, places or objects that I feel attached to

We are all born with an instinctive alarm system that triggers when our survival is threatened. When we are very small, this alarm system is activated when we find ourselves in 'strange' situations. Our alarm goes off making us feel anxious and we react with behaviour that maximises our chance of survival which is finding and getting close to a protective adult. This is usually achieved by behaviour such as following, clinging and crying. These behaviours are called attachment behaviours. Over time, as we mature, our attachment behaviours change; they become modified by our experiences and by the way in which our protective adult reacts to us. We learn how to deal with strange situations and to manage anxious feelings without immediately needing to get physically next to someone we trust. Many people have certain objects (e.g. coats, money, keys, blanket) and places (e.g. bed, home) which help them to cope with feeling anxious, but being close to people who we feel can protect us and who we trust remains important throughout our life.

Living with dementia can bring moments that feel like a strange situation again and research findings suggest that, in later life, early attachment relationships, such as those we make with our parent(s), can be a valuable resource to help us to cope when attachment bonds become disrupted (Browne and Shlosberg 2006, p.1).

Early important studies were conducted by Miesen (1993, 1997), who was interested in the concept of 'parental fixation' to help our understanding of the emotional world of people with dementia. It is becoming increasingly observed now that some people living with dementia demonstrate behaviour related to parent fixation, such as calling out and searching for parents, enquiring as to how their parents are, and asking to go home (Browne and Shlosberg 2006).

Behaviours like these then may be telling us that the person is feeling anxious and alarmed and that they are unable to calm themselves down and so are looking for someone to make them feel safe and secure (the attachment figure). If the person cannot find an attachment figure they may well adopt an alternative strategy which is to talk about somebody they trust or go to a place where they feel safe or to physically hold on to a symbolic object as a way of calming themselves down.

In this section you should record those attachment figures, stored in the person's memory and physically available, including people, pets, objects, places, which seem to be important to help them feel safe, secure and calm:

1. people such as family members, close friends – remember that these can be attachment figures even if the relationship between them is not warm and supportive

2. staff members, other professionals (e.g. a key worker, chaplain, social worker)

3. people now dead (e.g. parents, siblings, old friends, children who died or are no longer children because they grew up)

4.   pets who the person talks about a lot, or tries to find

5.   objects (e.g. soft toys, coat, handbag, clock)

6.   places or pictures of places (e.g. home, parents' home, favourite place)

7.   times in the person's life that are good to talk about because they become less anxious and alarmed when they revisit them (in their imagination).

Here is an example of how you might fill in the Attachment section of the Lifestyle and Future Wishes Template.

People, places or objects that I feel attached to

Yvette spends most afternoons saying that she wants to go home.

James worries about his mum when he gets tired.

Moira is very attached to her two cats (soft toys) who she calls 'my boys', she keeps them with her most of the time.

Bill is very attached to Maggie and likes to sit next to her and hold hands. He likes being in bed with her too.

What I do and what I need to help me feel close to them

For Yvette: 'I stand by the door and try to get home.'

For James: 'I like to stay close to staff when I am worried about my mum.'

For Moira: 'I keep my boys with me most of the time.'

For Bill: 'I like to be with Maggie. If I wake in the night and she's not there I go and find her.'

In this section, any person (such as a close friend or family member) or object (such as a soft toy) that clearly helps the person with dementia to maintain their 'hold' on the world and to feel safe should be recorded. Being 'with' a significant attachment figure or object often has the effect of keeping the person with dementia feeling safe, secure and calm.

If the person you are profiling talks about home or parents or is physically attached to a particular person or object, this should be written in this section.

Sexuality and attachment are often linked and it may be that the person being profiled wishes to openly express his or her need for intimacy. Sexual needs might be expressed verbally or through actions and behaviour; or the person may wish to keep their personal issues regarding sexuality private. For this reason, there is not a specific section in the template for recording information about sexuality and sexual needs. However, ignoring this important aspect of a person is not appropriate if the principles of person-centred care are to be applied fully to the process of enriched care planning. This is a delicate area, and needs to be approached sensitively and in a way that is acceptable to and manageable for the person. Many people feel that their sexuality and their sexual needs are not things to be discussed openly. So, talking about sexuality is not something that we should rush into before getting to know people and direct questions are not always appropriate. Many people have secrets about their sexuality that they will not want to share e.g. married people who have had affairs all their lives, homosexuals who have never 'come out'. In many cases we find out more about a person's needs from their behaviour than by asking direct questions. On the other hand it is important to signal to people that it is alright to talk about their sexuality and sexual needs.

Sexuality is not much to do with 'sex'. It is part of who we are; how we see ourselves; how we dress; how we are in our relationships with other people and the feelings we have about other people. Sexuality can be expressed through jokes and innuendo, flirting and romantic attachments. Understanding and encouraging this kind of sexuality is relatively easy for caregivers. Stirling Dementia Services Development Centre has produced a CD to help carers to work effectively and appropriately with sexuality.

Despite old age, dementia, physical frailty and loss of previous sexual partners, many people wish to remain sexually active. Engaging in sexual relationships can bring love, intimacy and closeness as well as physical release and these things can contribute a great deal to older people's general well-being (Wallace 1992). Challenging and uncomfortable though it may be for carers, it is important to understand that age and disability do not obliterate a person's desire for sex. Sexual intercourse, masturbation, caressing and touching commonly take place in family and care homes, and cause a great deal of concern, discomfort and distress for carers. This is often reflected in the use of words such as 'inappropriate', 'challenging', 'grabbing', 'groping' and 'obscene' when describing sexual behaviour (Nagaratnam and Gayagay 2002). For person-centred practice, we need to make accurate observations and use non-judgemental and respectful language to describe sexual activity.

The involvement of family members in discussions of sexuality and sexual needs is another delicate area. While family members may have strong feelings and opinions about the sexual activity of their father, mother, husband or wife, their agenda and their interests are different and separate. The person may not wish their family to be involved in discussion or decisions about their sexual activity.

Your own relationship with the person and your age, gender and even your own issues relating to sexuality are all relevant too. Talking to a relative stranger may or may not be easier than talking to a familiar person; a woman may be more comfortable talking to another woman; an older person may or may not wish to discuss their sexual preferences or needs with a much younger person; a heterosexual person may object to discussing sexuality with a gay person and a gay person may prefer to talk to another gay person.

There are no quick fix, fit all solutions here. But here is some guidance that may be helpful:

- Think about your own feelings.

- Be aware that feelings for family members can run high.

- Approach each situation 'case by case'.

- Be open-minded.

- Be aware that you can and should 'manage' risk but you cannot eliminate it.

- Try to limit damage when you make decisions – the remedy to a problem shouldn't be more harmful than letting it be.

- A key issue and responsibility for carers is to protect vulnerable adults; ask the question 'is this person vulnerable in this situation?'

- Know the Mental Capacity Act (2005) and abide by its principles.

- Seek guidance and support from outside experts such as the Advocacy Service.

Be aware that promoting an understanding of a person's sexuality can bring benefits such as having a healthy self-image, psychological refuelling and re-energizing, an outlet for personal anxieties, and a means of preventing social disengagement and avoiding depression (Heath 1999).

For a person who is less able to use words to express needs, their sexual behaviour may be an expression of a very strong and basic need and this is relevant for inclusion in the Lifestyle and Future Wishes Profile provided the person and/or their advocate is in agreement.

Remember that, at this profiling stage of the enriched care planning process, you are concerned with understanding and describing 'the person' rather than writing down problems or finding potential solutions. Here is a case example to help illustrate how you might write about sexuality.

Jim and Jean live in the same nursing home and both have dementia and although they are both married to other people, they apparently no longer recognise their spouses. Both really enjoy each other's company, and their relationship has become closer. They walk around the home holding hands and occasionally cuddling, but now Jim tries to steer Jean into a more private place and has been noticed to touch her in an obviously sexual manner.

For Jim, in the section entitled 'People, places or objects that I feel attached to' you might write something like 'I feel attached to Jean'. Underneath 'What I do and what I need to help me feel close to them' you could say 'I hold Jean's hand and cuddle her. This sometimes makes me want to have more intimate contact with her.' For Jean, you might write 'I am attached to Jim'; 'I need to be allowed to enjoy his company and to hold hands only when this is comfortable for me.'

This information can then be considered, along with all the information from the Life Story, Personality, Health, Capacity for Doing, Cognitive Ability and Life at the Moment Profiles, when you come to the 'identifying needs' stage of the care planning process which in turn would be incorporated into Jean and Jim's care plans.

Responding helpfully and ethically to the sexual needs of older people in group care settings requires mature, open and honest teamwork within a setting where comfortable and safe discussions about sexual issues can be supported. Strategies for responding to sexual needs in group care settings still need to be thought through and researched much more widely in the UK. We have been slow to move forward in the care sector, because of the taboo around the subject of sex and older people.

My spirituality

Spirituality does not mean the same as being religious, although many people engage in religious activity as part of their own spirituality. While not every human being is religious, we are all spiritual in some way or other; we all have our own way of finding meaning and purpose in life and people who have dementia have just as much need, if not more, to continue to do this. Rather like sexuality, this can for some people be a very private area.

It is not always easy to make a clear distinction between general well-being and spiritual well-being. One way to think about the difference is that general well-being is about day-to-day life – comfort, security, social inclusion and occupation – while spiritual well-being is about feeling at peace with wider questions such as the meaning of life, accepting the life we have lived and understanding the 'product' of our life. There are times when you can see in a person's body language that they are connecting with the world on another plane, out of the mundane trend of life. The Royal College of Psychiatrists offers helpful guidance to anybody needing to explore spirituality. Contact details are included in the list of useful resources at the back of this book.

It is always a good idea to consider whether there might be a spiritual aspect to what is happening for the person you are profiling, particularly if they seem troubled or distressed:

- Could an understanding of their spiritual beliefs or religious background help to understand their distress?

- Could it be that they are frightened about what might happen to them after death? (e.g. meeting up with a violent father)

- Can they talk about how they responded to troubles in the past? If they took a spiritual approach, might this be helpful now?

- Would it help to involve a chaplain, or someone from their faith community?

- Would discussion of their spiritual beliefs and needs with them, or with family members, be helpful?

- Might more contact with important spiritual symbols be helpful? (e.g. placing significant images where they can see them)

Questions that might help you to explore spirituality include:

- Are there any things that you like to look at, touch or hold that have special meaning or that feel important to you? (e.g. in nature, buildings, images, statues, the cross or other medals and pendants)

- How do you feel about the future?

- Do you experience a feeling of belonging and being valued for who you are, a sense of safety, respect and dignity? (Bruce 1998)

Use the 'My spirituality' box to write down key things that come up during these conversations. For example:

> Yvette definitely has a sense of spirituality. She feels connected to other people especially loved ones who have died such as her mother and father. She feels her purpose in life is to carry on goodness in the human race and she is happy that she has done her best to achieve this. Yvette sees flowers as representations of 'goodness' and would like more of them in her room.

> James says he is not religious but that he has had a purpose in life to continue on the family line which he has done. He does not really value or like talking about spirituality.

Future wishes

This is where you record what the person wants and doesn't want to happen if they become unable to communicate. This part of the profiling process can only be undertaken at a time when the person is able and willing to discuss their future wishes.

If the person you are profiling is unable or unwilling to discuss their future wishes, you should find out if they have made their wishes known in writing or verbally to anybody else and record this. You will also need to find out if the person has appointed anybody to make decisions on their behalf. This person might be referred to as an 'attorney'. The attorney only takes up their role if the person who appointed them (the donor) loses mental capacity and becomes unable to make or communicate their own decisions. If you think this is the case, you should contact the Office of the Public Guardian and take advice about how to proceed.

If you find yourself giving care or support to a person who cannot communicate their own wishes and you have not got any information about their wishes or the arrangements they have made, you are bound by law to act in what you believe to be their best interests. Knowing about the person's life story, lifestyle, personality, health, cognitive support needs and capacity for doing will equip you well to act in their best interests.

If the person being profiled indicates that there are medical treatments that they would not want in the future, you must help them to discuss this with their doctor or another senior person and to make a written statement so that everybody is absolutely clear. The statement needs to be signed and dated and witnessed and ideally entitled 'Advance directive, refusing treatment'. This statement is legally binding, meaning that the treatment cannot be lawfully given. However, the legal binding only applies to wishes about medical treatment.

Because issues of consent, capacity and communication can be complex, you and the person you are profiling should seek advice and support as you tackle the job of talking about and writing down future wishes. A good place to start is the Directgov website which is the official government website for citizens. The information and services available on the website are provided by a variety of UK government departments. Information about how to make a Living Will, which is sometimes called an Advance Decision or an Advance Directive can be accessed under the 'government, citizens and rights' section. If you are not comfortable using the internet, you can contact Age Concern or Mind and ask for a leaflet to be sent out to you. Contact details are included in the list of useful resources at the back of this book.

The Future Wishes page of the template provided with this best practice guide is a tool for helping you to talk about future wishes. A record of future wishes (UNLESS IT REFERS TO A WISH TO REFUSE ALL OR SOME FORMS OF MEDICAL TREATMENT) is not legally binding but health professionals will want to take it into account when deciding on a course of action. Family and friends might also want to use it as evidence of the person's wishes.

You will see that the second page of the template is divided into six parts:

- Please take into account these lifestyle preferences.

- I would be happy to accept the following additional treatments/support.

- I would prefer not to accept the following treatments/support.

- I want the following person/people to be consulted about my treatment/support at the time such decisions need to be made.

- I have/have not made an Advance Directive or Living Will.

- I have/have not appointed someone as an 'attorney' to make decisions on my behalf.

Please take into account these lifestyle preferences

This is an important reminder for anybody involved in providing care for the person to respect that person's lifestyle when they are making decisions about or providing care. There is space to write those very important things that the person you are profiling would not want to be overlooked were they unable to communicate their wishes. For example, being vegetarian or belonging to a particular religious group.

Treatments and support

You should be very clear about what these are.

Treatments include:

- surgery

- drugs

- cardiac resuscitation

- blood transfusion.

Support includes:

- being washed, bathed, fed, dressed.

I would be happy to accept the following additional treatments/support

This section is where you record what the person clearly wants and under what circumstances. For example:

'If I become immobile and I cannot communicate my wishes, I want to be kept comfortable, clean and pain free.'

'I would be happy to accept pain killers if my carers think I am in pain.'

'I want to be washed and dressed by my carers if I am happy and co-operative when they are helping me.'

'I am happy to be fed if I show that I want the food and that I am enjoying the food being given to me.'

'If I am physically strong and well and I suddenly stop breathing, I do want to be resuscitated.'

I would prefer not to accept the following treatments/support

Here is where you write down what the person has clearly indicated they do not want and under what circumstances. For example:

'I do not want my carers to handle me if this makes me upset.'

'If I develop a terminal condition, I do not want invasive surgery.'

'If I am bed-bound and physically weak and I stop breathing, I do not want to be resuscitated.'

'Under no circumstances do I want a blood transfusion.'

I want the following person/people to be consulted about my treatment/support at the time such decisions need to be made

The names of the person or people to be consulted about treatment/support at the time such decisions need to be made, should be recorded here. These must be people named by the person being profiled. If the person does not want to name anybody, then this should be respected.

I have/have not made an Advance Directive or Living Will

If the person has a previously drawn up Advance Directive or Living Will you need to state this and give details of where it is kept. For ease of access, it might also be a good idea to copy wishes from the person's Living Will onto this template, if the person is happy for you to do this and, of course, if these are still their wishes.

I have/have not appointed someone as an 'attorney' to make decisions on my behalf

Similarly, if an attorney has been appointed write down who this is and where the paperwork is kept. If an attorney has not been appointed and the person is capable of appointing one you should ask them if they would like help to sort this out. It is strongly recommended that we all appoint an attorney to make decisions on our behalf in the event of incapacity.

An attorney can only be appointed by the person when the person has the capacity to make such arrangements and decisions. It is possible to appoint different attorneys for different roles and there is space in this section to record the names of more than one attorney should this be needed. An attorney is usually a family member or friend who takes on the role of making decisions about the person's property, financial and other affairs and welfare when the person becomes incapable of making their own decisions. When this happens, the person's mental capacity needs to be assessed and the Power of Attorney applied for through the Office of the Public Guardian and the Court of Protection. Contact details are included in the list of useful resources at the back of this book.

Finally, in this section, there is space to write down whether or not the person's Lasting Power of Attorney (LPA) has been registered with the the Office of the Public Guardian and where original documents and copies are held.

IDENTIFYING AND DOCUMENTING NEEDS FROM THE LIFESTYLE AND FUTURE WISHES PROFILE

Identifying needs

Identifying needs here involves linking those aspects of the person's unique profile that they need help to maintain or see through in relation to their lifestyle and future wishes. You will need to look through the profile carefully and try to identify those things that are crucial for the person's well-being. These might include:

- eating habits
- favourite colours
- dressing routine
- having support for work-like activities
- how the individual expresses attachment, sexual and spiritual needs
- what the person wants if they become unable to communicate.

Examples of how these things might be relevant to needs:

- Eating habits – the person may have a set routine for eating which, if not maintained, causes them to become unsettled and upset.

- Favourite colours – knowing these can be used to promote the person's sense of worth and identity.

- Dressing routine – not knowing how the individual likes to go about this can get them off to a bad start with repercussions through the rest of the day.

- Having support for work-like activities – the person's need for occupation will be better met if their carer(s) understand and support the type of work-like activities that the person initiates themselves.

- How the individual expresses attachment, sexual and spiritual needs – knowing about these will prevent behaviour from becoming or being perceived as unacceptable.

- What the person wants if they become unable to communicate – this will guide the carer(s) through what is best to do in the interests of the person if communication is difficult.

Documenting needs

Having identified what is important for the person, you will now need to reflect this in what you write in the three working templates:

- Brief Profile Sheet
- Key Information Sheet
- The Enriched Care Plan.

Brief Profile Sheet

There is a space in the second section of the Brief Profile Sheet 'Important Issues Relating to my Lifestyle and Future Wishes'. There is only room to briefly summarise the very important things, and you will need to talk to the person and/or their family to decide what these are. The most important things are likely to be related to culture. For example, you would write in this section if the person is vegetarian or follows a particular faith or sect such as Jehovah's Witness, Roman Catholic, Hindu or Muslim. If the person has a strong wish about what should and shouldn't happen to them in the future (e.g. about resuscitation) and if they have made an Advance Directive and appointed an attorney this also should be recorded here.

Key Information Sheet

There may be people who have come up during profiling lifestyle and future wishes that the person may want you to contact, regularly or in emergencies, on their behalf. This section is entitled 'People that I may wish to contact'. You would record the name and contact details of the person's attorney if they have appointed one.

The other section of relevance in the Key Information Sheet is further down the page and entitled 'Important information that I want people involved in my care to know about'. Again, if anything has come up during profiling of lifestyle and future wishes that the person feels is very important for others to know about, it can be recorded here, for example that a Living Will has been made and where it is kept.

The Enriched Care Plan

The end product, the Enriched Care Plan, will be drawn from all the profiling that you do in relation to life story, lifestyle and future wishes, personality, health, capacity for doing, cognitive ability and life at the moment. There are just three columns in the plan. On the left hand side is the column entitled 'I need'. The middle column is headed 'My carers will'. The right hand column is for recording a date for review.

At this stage in the enriched care planning process, you only need write in the 'I need' column in relation to needs arising from lifestyle and future wishes. As already said, these needs will be things that make or break the person's day, things that are important *to* the person.

Here are some examples of how you might document needs in relation to lifestyle and future wishes within the Enriched Care Plan:

I need

My eating routine to be supported:

- no breakfast
- a biscuit and coffee at 9.00 am
- main meal at 5.00 pm
- snack at 10.00 pm.

To be offered clothes to wear that are blue which is my favourite colour.

To get dressed after I have had my biscuit and coffee.

To be validated and supported by staff when I try to help to lay the table.

To have flowers in my room.

To be supported to keep my friendship with Jim.

To be helped to find my own space again when Jim becomes over-amorous.

SUMMARY

- A lifestyle is the way in which a person lives, usually affected by the wider cultural context.

- If the individual's cultural essence is not understood and respected, there is a risk that behaviour will be judged as 'challenging' or 'inappropriate'.

- Enriched care planning takes account of lifestyle issues that are relevant and important to the individual.

- These include food and drink, clothes, daily living activities, work-like activities, relaxing and social activities, personal attachment figures or objects and spirituality.

- As part of the enriched care planning process, it may be appropriate for you to help the person you are profiling to think about and write down their future wishes.

- Identifying needs in relation to lifestyle and future wishes involves identifying those aspects of the person's unique profile that they need help to maintain or see through in relation to their lifestyle and future wishes.

- The Enriched Care Plan will include actions that carers need to take in order to respect the person's lifestyle and future wishes.

Chapter 4

Personality

Personality has been described as '…that pattern of characteristic thoughts, feelings, and behaviours that distinguishes one person from another and that persists over time and situation' (Phares 1991). It is logical then to go on and say that dementia will not and cannot affect any two people in the same way, because their personalities are actually different. This has been completely overlooked in old culture practice where 'behaviour' has more often than not been attributed entirely to 'the dementia'.

Having dementia brings many changes in a person's day-to-day living experience. These changes might include finding oneself in a 'being cared for' relationship and possibly living in an unfamiliar situation with a group of unknown others.

> Noise or motion feels like an egg beater in my head, scrambling what is in there and putting a static sound or visual screen over what is coming in. It is as if I have lost the filter in my brain, to focus on one thing out of many. Sounds become a 'hubbub' and I can't make out what people are saying to me. (Bryden 2005, p.114)

Living in such a changed world would without a doubt give rise to strong feelings within any human being which in turn would influence their reaction. It is important to understand though that the reactions between different people will be different because we all have our own unique personality.

Currently, the most well-researched way of looking at and understanding personality is to use the five factor model of personality (McCrae and Costa 2003). The five factors or dimensions are neuroticism, extraversion, openness to experience, agreeableness and conscientiousness. These dimensions are thought to be stable across a lifespan and seem to have a physiological base (McCrave and Costa 2003). The theory is that our personality is made up of the combination of our tendency towards each of these traits. For example, one person might tend greatly towards extraversion but not towards agreeableness while for another person this might be the other way around: a strong tendency towards agreeableness but not towards extraversion. Such combinations, and in this example I have only combined two dimensions and not the entire five, are likely to result in very different reactions to the same situation.

It is often said that dementia causes a change of personality but there is little or no research to support or oppose this view. Certainly, having a diagnosis of dementia has been observed to change behaviour but this is not the same as personality and there are many reasons to cause a person to behave 'out of character'. Our position on this, at the time of writing, is that it is important to work with the firm belief that all people, including people who have dementia, do have a personality and that it is good practice in delivering person-centred care to find out about this.

Consider this true case scenario, set in the lounge of a nursing home, to illustrate the point:

A male nurse has been hit by Alex, a patient on the ward who has dementia. At the time of the incident, the nurse is administering lunchtime medication to residents in the lounge area. Old culture thinking would label Alex as 'aggressive', the rationale being 'he has dementia and is therefore aggressive'. What is missing here is any understanding of Alex's personality. He is actually a very sensitive man who acts on his feelings. He is reactive and easily bothered by what is happening around him. Alex is also extravert and this means he is physically active, adventurous and assertive. Furthermore, he is old fashioned, conservative in the way he sees things with fairly fixed ideas about what is right and what is wrong. Finally, Alex tends to act before he thinks; he has a tendency to be impulsive. What Alex saw when the nurse was administering medication in the lounge was a strong young man towering over a frail, elderly lady in a threatening way. His dementia may have caused him to misperceive what he saw but his personality tailored his behaviour – he was trying to protect the vulnerable lady. In an old culture setting, Alex might be medicated, segregated and avoided in response to his behaviour. A person-centred care team would be more aware of all the factors influencing behaviour including personality and manage his care accordingly.

Some people who have dementia may find it difficult to communicate in words about their own personality and so it may be helpful to involve a friend or family member, but this presents some problems. There may be differences between how the personality of a person with dementia was perceived by others before the onset of dementia, and how it is perceived now. Furthermore, these may be similar or different to how the person perceives themselves. For example, the way in which a daughter perceives her mother's personality will very likely be different to how that woman (who happens also to be a mother) perceives herself.

When profiling personality as part of the enriched care planning process, all perspectives are relevant. In the first instance, the perspective should come directly from the person who should be given the opportunity to describe and talk about their own personality. The enriched care planning Personality Template provides a framework taken from the five factor model as a structure for thinking and talking about personality.

USING THE PERSONALITY PROFILING TEMPLATE

This template can be used to generate discussion with the person being profiled and/or their carer(s), or to help you to think about the person if you are completing the template on their behalf. You can expect to mark the 'x' for each box in a different place each time. In some boxes, it will veer to the left; in others it may be in the middle or veering more to the right. Each box represents one of the five factors or dimensions which are neuroticism, extraversion, openness to experience, agreeableness and conscientiousness. It is best to use the words provided in the boxes rather than the names of the actual dimensions. You may need to get more information from other people and/or through observation, in which case you will draw your profile from observing the person, spending time with them and talking to other people who know the person well.

There are five boxes, one for each of the dimensions described above which make up the Personality Template. Use the template to help you to talk with the person and any others involved to draw up a unique profile. Use the space underneath to make comments: to quote what the person says about themselves, or to describe what you have observed or what has been said to you by others about this person's personality.

The words used for this template are intended to generate discussion but you should feel free to use different words if you need to so that they have meaning for the person you are talking with. Invite the person to decide where they are on each line and/or write key words and phrases that the person and/or others uses in the boxes. In many ways, the process that you go through, the discussions you have and the relationship that develops between you and the person you are profiling is more important than the end result piece of paper.

Box 1: Sensitive, nervous vs. secure, confident

This box relates to 'neuroticism' in the five factor theory which is a rather unpleasant term usually associated with a psychiatric label. However, what it actually means is negativity or nervousness. A person who sees themselves as more sensitive and nervous is likely to be less emotionally in control than one who sees themselves as more confident and secure. The nervous, sensitive type tends to be reactive; more easily upset by what is happening around them and to experience more frequently feelings of anxiety and sadness. A person who is more confident and secure on the other hand is not so easily provoked.

Examples of questions you might ask

- When you were little, did you ever feel nervous?
- Were you bold and confident?
- Have you changed much since then?
- Would you say now that you are very nervous, or not really?
- Do you feel nervous/confident a lot or just sometimes?
- So, would you say you are in the middle somewhere?
- Or definitely on the nervous/confident end of things?

Box 2: Outgoing, energetic vs. shy, withdrawn

This relates to the 'extraversion' dimension of the five factor theory and contrasts an outgoing, energetic personality with a more withdrawn type. Extraverts are independent and active in nature; they can be very frank and assertive and they enjoy socialising. Introverts tend to be shy, reserved and less sociable.

Examples of questions you might ask

- Would you say you are a shy person?
- Are you the type of person who is outgoing?
- Do you like mixing with other people?
- It sounds to me that you are a bit of an introvert; shall we put the x at that end of the scale?

Box 3: Inventive, curious vs. cautious, conservative

This relates to the 'openness to experience' dimension of the five factor theory. A person who is open to experience has a good imagination; likes to experience new and different things; has broad interests; and is liberal. In contrast, those with low openness to experience, sometimes known as 'preservers' are conventional, conservative and prefer familiarity.

Examples of questions you might ask

- Do you like each day to be different or do you prefer a nice steady routine?

- Are you the type of person who has lots of new ideas?

- Would you say you're a bit whacky, or rather conventional?

- Are you a curious or cautious type?

Box 4: Friendly, compassionate vs. competitive, outspoken

This relates to the 'agreeableness' dimension of the five factor theory and is linked to traits of friendliness, caring and emotional support versus competitiveness, self-centeredness, outspokenness, spitefulness and jealousy. Agreeable people can be described as kind, sympathetic and warm.

Examples of questions you might ask

- Are you the warm and cuddly type?

- Do other people see you as friendly and agreeable, or are you more of an outspoken type?

- Do you feel caring or more competitive towards other people?

- Are you the jealous type?

Box 5: Efficient, organised vs. easy-going, carefree

This relates to the 'conscientiousness' dimension of the five factor theory. The more conscientious a person is the more competent, dutiful, orderly, responsible and thorough they are (McCrae and Costa 2003). People who have this trait are able to control their impulses far more than a more flexible and easy-going type who is likely to be a bit carefree and more impulsive.

Examples of questions you might ask

- Are you an organised person, do you like a timetable?

- Do you often feel responsible for getting things done?

- Are you a stickler for detail or more slapdash?

- How do you cope when the plan changes, are you quite flexible?

Profiling personality should be fun and a positive experience for all concerned. Knowing yourself does not depend on memory and so the person you are profiling should be able to tell you a lot about this. Remember, the template is just there as a guide, it isn't important to put a cross on each line so leave this out if it feels uncomfortable. What is important is the whole 'getting to know you' process which can be done individually, in a group and certainly over a period of time.

IDENTIFYING AND DOCUMENTING NEEDS FROM THE PERSONALITY PROFILE

Identifying needs

Identifying needs in relation to personality requires you to know about individual characteristics that may affect the person's well-being in the current situation. Look back over the profile and, if possible together with the person, identify anything important that would be relevant now. Important information might include extremes of:

- nervousness

- shyness

- curiosity

- outspokenness

- wanting to be organised, in control.

The reason that these are more likely to be of relevance in this context is because these characteristics can often be perceived as 'part of the dementia' or as 'difficult' or 'challenging' behaviour. Understanding that they are part and parcel of who the person is makes a person-centred approach easier.

Examples of how these things might be relevant to needs:

- Nervousness – the person may need regular reassurance to prevent their anxiety from escalating.

- Shyness – the person may do better in a one-to-one situation; they may not enjoy being put under pressure socially.

- Curiosity – this can make a person active and determined.

- Outspokenness – can be perceived as hostility.

- Wanting to be organised, in control – the person may become anxious and upset if this aspect of their personality is not supported.

Documenting needs

Having identified what is important for the person, you will now need to reflect this in what you write in the three working templates:

- Brief Profile Sheet
- Key Information Sheet
- The Enriched Care Plan.

Brief Profile Sheet

There is a space in the third section of the Brief Profile Sheet 'Important Issues Relating to my Personality'. There is only room to briefly summarise the very important things, and you will need to talk to the person and/or their family to decide what these are. Examples of what you might write here include: 'James is a blunt, outspoken personality and always has been, he does not intend to hurt people's feelings' or 'Yvette is very shy and prefers not to be pressurised into joining in with group activities.'

Key Information Sheet

The section of relevance in the Key Information Sheet is further down the page and is entitled 'Important information that I want people involved in my care to know about'. If anything has come up during profiling of personality that the person feels is very important for others to know about, it can be recorded here. For example if a person is very nervous and needs lots of reassurance, or adventurous and curious and needs space and time to live this out.

The Enriched Care Plan

The end product, the Enriched Care Plan, will be drawn from all the profiling that you do in relation to life story, lifestyle and future wishes, personality, health, capacity for doing, cognitive ability and life at the moment. There are just three columns in the plan. On the left hand side is the column entitled 'I need'. The middle column is headed 'My carers will'. The right hand column is for recording a date for review.

At this stage in the enriched care planning process, you only need write in the 'I need' column in relation to needs arising from personality. As already said, these needs will be things that make or break the person's day, things that are important *to* the person.

Examples of what you might include in the 'I need' column:

- support from my carer(s) to hold my own in social situations

- to feel in control by having my living space neat and orderly

- people to know I am a blunt person but this does not mean that I do not like them.

SUMMARY

- Dementia cannot affect any two people in the same way, because their personalities are different.

- In old culture practice 'behaviour' has more often than not been attributed entirely to the effects of dementia without consideration of personality.

- For person-centred practice, it is important to work with the firm belief that all people, including people who have dementia, do have a personality.

- The enriched care planning Personality Template provides a framework taken from the five factor model as a structure for thinking and talking about personality.

- Identifying needs in relation to personality requires you to know about individual characteristics that may affect the person's well-being in the current situation.

- The Enriched Care Plan will identify needs in relation to the person's unique personality that need to be taken into account in their current day-to-day living experience.

Chapter 5

Health

The impact of physical and mental health problems can often be lessened and yet these problems, when they arise for a person who has dementia, are sometimes ignored or seen as part of having dementia. This was certainly the case for Barry, one of the patients on a long-stay dementia care ward who had always, despite his poor mobility and difficulty speaking, smiled a lot. Nobody could remember exactly when, but it came to be noticed that he wasn't smiling any more. The ward team put this down to 'the dementia' assuming he had generally deteriorated. We were all very upset and shocked when it eventually became apparent that he had broken his hip.

A person who has dementia may not be able to report on or adequately manage their own physical or mental health issues and the risk of treatable health problems being missed can be high. For this reason, physical and mental health should be routinely profiled. For anybody new to a care setting, the profile should be completed as soon as possible. This part of the enriched care planning process involves consideration of the person's physical and mental health from their perspective in addition to information from health assessments and reports that have already been done and identification of any current health issues that need to be assessed further.

Profiling health should be something that the person with dementia is fully involved in. Under the Mental Capacity Act (2005), you are required to work with the person who has dementia assuming that he or she does have the capacity to make their own decisions unless found otherwise. This means, that when you are helping the person to profile and manage their own health, you have an obligation to take all practicable steps to help the person make his or her own decisions. Mental capacity is not a static thing – a person may have the capacity to make a decision about one situation (e.g. whether or not to take pain killers for a headache) but not another (eg whether or not to have surgery for prostate cancer). Mental capacity can also change or fluctuate depending on factors such as how tired the person is feeling, how physically well or unwell they are and how well information is being presented to them.

Mental capacity is assessed in relation to single decisions using these criteria:

- Can the person understand information relevant to the decision, including understanding the likely consequences of making, or not making the decision?

- Can they retain this information for long enough to make the decision?

- Can they use and weigh up the information to arrive at a choice?

- Can they communicate their decision in any way?

If the person lacks capacity, the onus then falls on the person who has a duty of care to act in that person's best interests. If the person lacks capacity you should check whether he or she has appointed an attorney to make health-related decisions on their behalf. There is more about this in the 'future wishes' section of Chapter 3.

Acting in an individual's best interests will involve using a combination of verbal and non-verbal communication and sensitive observation to find out as much as possible about the health issue being profiled. You should also involve a family member or friend who knows the person and who also has their interests at heart, to work with you and any other appropriate staff or carers. It is good practice to ask the person who has dementia if they would like another person to speak for them, and if so, who.

In care settings where nursing and medical care is being provided, information relating to physical health such as body temperature, pulse rate and blood pressure may be required. The Health Template included with this good practice guide does not make provision for profiling these because they require a trained nurse or doctor. However, the nursing staff involved in the piloting of this enriched care planning process found it very easy to incorporate their own documentation with the Enriched Care Plan.

The information you record here is different from the information you record when completing the Lifestyle and Future Wishes Profile. Lifestyle is more to do with preferences – for example, preferring sweet food to savoury food, preferring tea to coffee or preferring cardigans to sweaters – whereas in the Health Profile the focus is more on functioning and what the person needs to maintain healthy functioning. If you do find that overlaps and repetitions are occurring during the profiling process, don't worry! This doesn't matter; the main reason for going through this profiling process is to get to know 'the person' and to be able to understand what their needs are and how to meet them.

Information is gathered during the health profiling process by finding out in detail about current health conditions and treatments; how the person copes with everyday basic daily living; any potential unmet physical or mental health needs; risks; pain and the person's preference for addressing dementia. This information can then be used to help the person to stay well as well as alerting the carer(s) when something is wrong. For example, something might be wrong if a person who normally eats three meals a day is now only eating very small amounts. However, for a person who only eats very small amounts there would be no cause for concern. Similarly, there would be no cause for concern for a person who has always stayed up late and slept on a settee to be doing the same in a care setting whereas this would be a concerning pattern for somebody who has always retired early and slept in a bed.

Another good reason for learning about the way in which the person engages with these daily living activities is so that the person's needs for staying engaged with them can be understood and met. These familiar living experiences keep us mobile and provide a source of comfort and a sense of purpose and identity. This being said we need to be always mindful of how different and unique each person is. While one person may fall back on familiar routines and habits to help them to cope with failing cognitive ability another may want or need a different routine. Most importantly, it is good practice to explore poor health as a potential cause of changed behaviour or of ill-being or distress and to give priority to this when you are planning or reviewing the person's care.

USING THE HEALTH PROFILING TEMPLATE

This is the most complex and the longest of all the enriched care planning templates. There are four pages in all. Page 1 is for recording general information about current health issues; medicine and tablets; weight; nicotine and alcohol intake. Pages 2 and 3 are for recording detailed information about the functions of eating a good diet, drinking enough fluids, communicating, moving about safely, going to the toilet, sleeping, seeing well, hearing well, and needs for healthy teeth and gums, heart and lungs, feet and skin. For each of these, there is a profile column where you write the current situation, a special needs column where the person's needs for maintaining their current situation should be recorded and the option to tick a specialist assessment tick box if you and/or the person you are profiling requests this. There are sections for recording information about pain and specific risks to health for the person at the end of Page 3. On Page 4 there is space to record information about mental health and well-being and about the person's memory problems, diagnosis and how they wish this information to be managed.

My current health issues include

This is where you can write down relevant information about the person's current health issues. These include long-term, known conditions that the person needs help to manage in order to stay well and healthy. In an older person, it is likely that there will be more than one health issue.

Asking a person to tell you about their current health issues is a very open question and it might be helpful to break the question down into easier questions about single body systems or body parts.

For example, do you have any illnesses to do with your:

- muscles?

- bones?

- eyes, ears, nose?

- heart and lungs?

- stomach?

- arms and legs?

- fingers and toes?

You could help the person to focus on each part of their body in turn, say, starting at the feet, asking if they have any pain or discomfort in that part, or whether they need any cream or tablets or other help for that part. Some carers have found that using pictures or a doll when communication is difficult can help to prompt the person to think and talk about different areas of their own body.

Retrieving information from medical documents such as medical notes, nursing notes and specialist reports will be important. This information, coupled with what the person and their family and friends can tell you, will greatly reduce the risk of missing important information.

The person you are profiling is entitled to have access to his or her medical notes and there is the option for a representative to request the information on their behalf. The Data Protection Act (1998, 2000) states that a patient or a nominated representative can submit a 'subject access request' in writing to their General Practitioner with the appropriate fee. Unless receipt of the information will cause serious harm to the physical or mental health of the person, they are entitled to receive a copy of their medical notes within twenty-one days. More information about this can be obtained from the Department of Health and the British Medical Association. Contact details are included in the list of useful resources at the back of this book.

These are the treatments I have

Any prescribed medicines or tablets or other treatments that the person you are profiling currently needs should be written down in this section. Knowing what all of these are relies more on memory than on feeling and so it may be appropriate to ask the person you are profiling if you can see their tablets/medicine and if there is anybody that helps them with medication. The person will probably be more than happy for you to consult other people about this but it is good practice to seek permission.

These are the medications, substances and situations that cause me to have an allergic reaction

It is most important that this section is filled in. If the person you are profiling is unable to tell you about their allergies or they can't provide you with enough detail you should, with their permission, find out from family, friends and previous medical records. Medications might include penicillin, substances might be certain perfumes or creams or metals such as silver or gold and situations might include dusty rooms, environments that house cats or other pets or times of the year when the pollen count is high.

Weight

You should record what the person with dementia answers here. However, if in your opinion, the person looks unhealthily underweight or overweight, it might be appropriate to explore this with them. If you feel there is a health risk, you might ask the person if they would mind being weighed so that you can monitor their weight.

Smoking and drinking

The purpose of finding out about whether the person who has dementia smokes and/or drinks alcohol is twofold. First to maintain the person's well-being; being deprived of cigarettes or alcohol might be detrimental. Second for health reasons, there may be risks for a person who smokes or drinks that should be known when prescribing other treatments or medications.

You will see that there is a column for the profile and another for special needs for each of the functions of eating, drinking, communicating, moving about using the toilet and sleeping. The profile column is where you record how the person functions at the current time in all of these. Any help that the person currently receives in order to perform these activities should be recorded in the special needs column. If you can, write who assessed this need and when and describe what the intervention is. For example 'Betty was assessed by the occupational therapist in June 2008 and she needs a plate guard for knife and fork meals.'

If the person is having difficulty with the any of the daily living activities, or is experiencing physical or emotional discomfort as a result of doing or not doing the activity, you should ask the person if they would like a specialist assessment. If the person has difficulty making a decision or communicating a decision about this you should make a decision in their best interests and communicate this to the person and any other significant family members or carer(s). There is a tick box for indicating a specialist referral in the far right hand column.

Eating

Record here how much the person needs to eat and when they eat as well as details of food they must have and food they must not have. This will be especially important if the person has food allergies or is diabetic.

This seems fundamental but can so easily be overlooked in care settings that are led by institutional routines. A recent example comes to mind where a man was moved from an old culture ward where he reportedly never ate breakfast. It came to light just a few weeks after the move that he did enjoy breakfast but that he liked to drink a cup of tea when he first got up and eat his breakfast about an hour later. The old culture ward routine had not allowed for this. He had been 'given' his breakfast every morning at the same time, but rarely ate it. The staff in the new specialist dementia unit allowed individuals to practise their own individual routines in the mornings so breakfast was provided to suit the person rather than the institution.

Special needs relate to needs that the person has in order to eat well. These needs might be in relation to the cutlery needed, the way the food is presented or in relation to the conditions under which the person eats well. For example, it may be that a teaspoon is easier for the person to eat from than a large spoon; that a plate guard is helpful; that the person needs their food to be cut up; or that they prefer to eat alone rather than in a group. Use the special needs column to write down any specialist assessments that the person has had before, or tick the tick box in the far right hand column if the person might benefit from a specialist assessment now.

Specialist assessments for eating are usually sought when a person is experiencing significant difficulties with eating. Such an assessment might be undertaken by a speech and language therapist, an occupational therapist, a nutritionist, dietician or a specialist nurse depending on the nature of the difficulty being experienced by the person and how the services in your area are organised. An initial assessment by a doctor and a referral from the doctor to the specialist might be required.

Eating difficulties include:

- Muscular or co-ordination problems:

  o with the face, mouth or throat causing the person to choke or have difficulty with chewing or swallowing food

  o with the arms and/or hands causing the person to have difficulty holding or manipulating eating utensils

  o with the arms and/or hands causing the person to have difficulty performing eating actions such as cutting, scooping and getting food to the mouth.

- Cognitive problems causing the person to have difficulty manipulating eating utensils or performing eating actions such as cutting, scooping and getting food to the mouth.

- Medical, social, psychological or cultural problems affecting the person's ability or desire to eat.

Drinking

Here you need to find out about how much and when the person needs to drink. In the above example, the morning cup of tea was an important part of the gentleman's routine in the morning and so more information about what type of drink he was used to drinking and at what times would have been helpful for the carer(s) to know about.

You may need to rely on observation to find out how well the person is faring with the routine that the care setting is imposing. Is the person drinking enough fluids? When are drinks made available, how are they made available and is the person drinking what is offered? The British Dietetic Association advises that the average adult should consume 2.5 litres of water per day. Of this, 1.8 litres – the equivalent of six to seven glasses of water per day – must be obtained directly from beverages. This should be increased during periods of hot weather or during and after periods of physical activity. Contact details for the British Dietetic Association are included in the list of useful resources at the back of this book.

For a person who has dementia, special needs for drinking might include the need to have fluids presented regularly; to have the drink placed in the person's hand; to be helped to start off drinking with verbal prompts; to drink from a special cup or to be given thickened fluids or fruit jelly as a way of keeping hydrated.

Make a note in the special needs column if the person has had a specialist assessment in the past in relation to drinking or fluid intake. For example 'John was assessed by the speech and language therapist in November 2007 and he needs to have his drinks thickened.' If you or the person being profiled thinks that a specialist assessment is needed you should indicate this in the far right hand tick box. As with eating, this type of assessment would most probably be undertaken by a speech and language therapist, specialist nurse or occupational therapist.

Drinking difficulties include:

- Muscular or co-ordination problems:

  o with the face, mouth or throat causing the person to choke on fluids or have difficulty with sipping, sucking or swallowing

  o with the arms and/or hands causing the person to have difficulty holding or manipulating drinking vessels such as cups

  o with the arms and/or hands causing the person to have difficulty reaching for or picking up drinking vessels.

- Cognitive problems causing the person to have difficulty manipulating drinking vessels or initiating or performing drinking actions such as reaching for, picking up, sipping, sucking or swallowing fluids.

- Medical, social, psychological or cultural problems affecting the person's ability or desire to drink.

Communicating

As we get older, our ability to communicate and our style of communication changes. Older people in general tend to slow down, needing more time to express themselves but also more time to process information and to respond. There may be other changes to do with the mechanics of speaking. Some older people find it less easy to use the muscles needed for speaking efficiently causing words to sound slurred. Chest conditions and general frailty can cause the voice to lose strength and this also can affect communication.

Having dementia can affect a person's ability to communicate in a number of different ways, compounding any pre-existing difficulties. Most importantly, every person is different, and while there are some common difficulties directly attributable to dementia, carers should do their best to know and understand what each individual person needs to be able to communicate with those around them.

Ideally, the person themselves should be invited to discuss their communication needs but, if this is difficult, you will need to ask family members and use your own experience of communicating with the person. It is important to remember that communication is not just about talking. As much as 90 per cent of communication is achieved through facial expression, gestures, body language, touch and tone of voice. So, non-verbal techniques that the person uses should be included here too. Use this section to flag up any unmet needs and to record information about the person's existing communication style and the help they need to communicate.

Start by finding out if the person *does* have any difficulty with words or any particular style of using words. These might include:

- difficulty physically speaking because of poor motor control

- difficulty understanding words, due to poor hearing or neurological damage

- word-finding difficulty

- losing track

- incoherent speech.

Any non-verbal methods that the person uses should be noted too. For example:

- waving and other gestures

- nodding

- smiling

- winking

- hugging or holding hands

- making eye contact

- calling out

- humming, singing

- making facial expressions.

Use the profile column to describe how the person currently communicates. For example 'Yvette speaks very quietly and takes a long time to respond when spoken to. She uses words well but sometimes loses track of what she is saying. Yvette enjoys waving to people she likes and holding hands with her friends when they are near her. She grimaces and spits when she is upset or angry.' Then write in the special needs column all the things that other people do to help. 'Yvette needs lots of time to respond and reminding when she loses track. She likes to be waved at and to be physically close to people she likes.'

Moving about

Moving about allows us to change and control our location in the world and human beings have a strong and natural drive to do this. Moving about independently includes walking, crawling; moving into and out of a bed or a chair; changing one's position in bed or in a chair; self-propelling in a wheelchair; and self-driving a vehicle. Assisted moving about would include being physically or cognitively supported when changing position or moving; being lifted or hoisted; being wheeled in a chair or driven in a vehicle in order to change position or location. It is good practice to encourage and support moving about – being prevented from moving about brings reactions of frustration and anger which can lead to physical and psychological ill health and ill-being.

In this section you should record as much as you can about how and when the person moves about; the locations they want or need to access; and any 'triggers' that cause them to want to change their location. For a person who moves about by walking, you should find the extent to which they are active and confident with walking; how much walking they do, indoors and outdoors; and whether they have certain times in the day or the night when they choose to walk about. It may be the case that the person has always been very active and that they need to walk around a lot. If the person being profiled is prone to periods of anxiety and disorientation causing them to move about, for example, wanting to go home in the afternoons, this should also be recorded here. Or it could be that the person is unable to move without help and therefore needs a 'moving about' routine to be initiated and managed for them by somebody else. In this case you may need to think about a specialist assessment and tick the far right hand column to indicate that this is needed.

If the person being profiled has limited mobility, it is still important to find out about how active and confident they feel with the way they move about; how much moving about they do; and whether they have certain times in the day or night when they want to move about. For example a person with a history of falls coming from home into a care setting may be observably slow, unsteady and struggling to get in and out of their chair or bed independently. If they have been moving about freely at home they will want to remain active, possibly at night as well if this has been their routine. In a case such as this, you would need to record this in the person's profile: 'Sarah moves around a lot during the day and sometimes at night despite being unsteady on her feet.' In her case, it would be good practice to suggest a specialist mobility assessment so that appropriate cognitive and physical support can be made available as part of her Enriched Care Plan.

The consequences of a care plan that focuses heavily on fall prevention and that limits rather than supports the person's own routine for moving about will do nothing for maintaining and improving physical and psychological health and well-being. Immobility itself brings substantial hazards. Moving about is crucial in the prevention of, for example, faecal impaction (and incontinence), deep vein thrombosis (and pulmonary embolism), and gravitational oedema (and skin ulceration) and also for preventing isolation which causes loneliness and depression (Young and Dinan 1994).

If the person has already been assessed and subsequently uses a walking aid such as a stick or a rollator or they use a wheelchair; or they need manual assistance for any part of their moving about routine, such as help out of bed or out of a chair; or they need cognitive support such as reminders or help to initiate and sustain a moving about routine this should be recorded as a special need.

Using the toilet

Going to the toilet is a vital and routine part of everyday living. Experiencing difficulty going to the toilet is distressing, uncomfortable, embarrassing and can make a person's life quite miserable. But, for many people who have dementia toileting problems are overlooked or ignored and almost even expected as part of having a diagnosis of dementia. Unmanaged or poorly managed problems related to going to the toilet can have a serious negative effect on a person's health and well-being. A person-centred approach is one where the physical care environment and the people working in it act to minimise any difficulties experienced by people who have dementia in relation to going to the toilet.

Using the enriched care planning approach will guide you and the person you are profiling through a process which will enable individualised support for going to the toilet. In this profiling stage, you will need to find out what the person's current pattern is for going to the toilet. This may be difficult and it may take some time. You may need to employ a number of different methods including talking to the person; observing them; accessing previous health records; and communicating with other carers such as family and friends.

Part of the profiling work here then will involve finding out how often the person normally goes to the toilet and when and how they are used to going to the toilet. For example, it could be that a person uses the toilet to urinate once or twice at night and after every meal during the day. Some people empty their bowels three times a day; while for others it may be three times a week. This is a normal range for human beings (Continence Foundation 2008) and it is important to find out what is 'usual' for the person you are profiling.

If the person is prone to constipation or other bowel or urinary problems, special preventative measures that they currently use to help should be recorded in the special needs column such as incontinence wear, oral remedies and creams; the need for reminding or prompting or accompanying; the need for practical help with clothing, wiping clean, washing hands and/or getting on and off the toilet; the need for clear visual cues such as signage, use of colour contrast to help the person see the toilet, the washbasin and other objects that the person uses during their toileting routine such as toilet paper or grab rails; or the need for help to find the toilet.

For example, in the profile column for somebody relatively independent you might write 'Mr Young uses the toilet independently. He uses the adapted toilet on the ground floor during the day and he needs a commode in his room at night.' In the special needs column you would record that he needs a raised toilet seat and rail in his daytime communal toilet facility and a commode in his room at night and you would not need to tick the specialist assessment box unless you or Mr Young felt it would be helpful to have a specialised assessment.

For somebody with more complex needs you might write in the profile column something like 'Mary has mobility problems and is sometimes disorientated. She is not able to use the toilet independently.' In the special needs column you might write 'Mary needs to be asked before each meal if she needs to use the toilet and accompanied to the toilet when she wants to go. Mary can manage to use the toilet on her own once she gets there but needs help to get back from the toilet. At night, Mary needs reminding to use the toilet before she goes to bed and for the door to her toilet to be left open with the light on.'

If the person you are profiling is currently experiencing difficulty or discomfort using the toilet it will be a priority in their care plan to have an assessment so that causes and potential solutions can be found. In this situation, you might be writing in the profile column something like 'John does not seem to be able to use the toilet during the day or at night which is leading to problems for him. He is upset when his clothing is wet or soiled and he does not like wearing a pad.' In the special needs column, you would write 'not yet known' and you would definitely tick the specialist assessment box, preferably with agreement from John.

It is good practice to avoid referring to the person as 'incontinent' verbally or in writing unless they have been formally diagnosed as such and even then, only when it is necessary and appropriate to do so. Incontinence means 'loss of control of passing urine or faeces' and is just one of a number of reasons why a person who has dementia might be experiencing problems using the toilet. Problems may arise from a poorly adapted environment (e.g. signage not clear, toilet not in view, seat too high or too low) or as a consequence of cognitive and/or physical impairment.

Problems associated with cognitive impairment include:

- Being unable to plan, initiate or sustain a toileting routine. This means that, for the person who is 'living in the moment', they will only think about the toilet when they actually need to use it. If the person has added difficulties such as limited mobility, or problems finding the toilet, they may well not get there in time.

- Being unable to complete the toileting routine, e.g. forgetting to wipe clean or wash after using the toilet which can lead to soiling of clothing.

- Being unable to recognise or distinguish the conventional places and objects associated with the toilet. This might cause the person to use a sink, cupboard or other receptacle as a toilet or to use substitutes for toilet paper.

Problems associated with physical impairment include:

- Poor mobility and/or limited range of movement making it difficult for the person to

    o   get out of their chair or bed to go to the toilet

    o   walk the distance to and from the toilet

    o   manage to get on and off the toilet

    o   manage their clothing through the toileting routine.

- Weakness of the muscles that control the bladder leading to 'stress incontinence' where urine leaks out.

- An overactive bladder resulting in the person feeling very little warning of the need to pass urine. This is called 'urgency' – when this happens, there may not be enough time to reach the toilet resulting in urine leaking.

- Enlarged prostate (in men only) which interferes with the flow of urine through the bladder causing difficulty passing water, or a 'jumpy' bladder triggering frequent trips to the toilet.

- Nocturia – needing to go to the toilet often at night. This can lead to bed wetting or 'enuresis'.

- Overflow incontinence which means that the person cannot stop their bladder from constantly dribbling, or continuing to dribble for some time after they have passed water.

- Anal sphincter damage causing the person to rush to the toilet as soon as the need is felt with often not enough time to get there or causing stools to leak out without the person realising this is happening.

- Diarrhoea which sometimes creates such extreme urgency that the person cannot get to the toilet in time.

- Constipation where the bowel becomes overloaded which causes amounts of faeces to break off and come away, usually without the person feeling that it is happening. Alternatively, the wall of the bowel is irritated by the hard stools and so produces more fluid and mucus, which then leaks out.

- Nerve injury or disease where damage stops the person getting the right messages when their rectum is full. Or the rectum may just empty automatically without feeling or control as soon as it fills.

A person who has dementia may have a combination of these problems which is why a proper assessment is important. A proper medical assessment as well as input from a specialist, such as an incontinence nurse or advisor and/or an occupational therapist or physiotherapist or even a combination of these professionals together, should be able to assess the problem(s) thoroughly in order to recommend the help and support needed to maximise the person's dignity, health and well-being.

Sleeping

The amount of sleep we each need, when and where we sleep and the conditions under which we sleep well or not are highly individual but sleeping too much or not enough can be a symptom or a cause of ill health. For people who have dementia, while sleep disturbance is a common experience (Passmore 2005), it is not necessarily a health issue. This section of the Health Template is designed to help you and the person you are profiling explore whether there are any health issues related to sleeping with a view to sorting them out.

One of the 'old culture' ideas that has led to institutionalisation of older people in some care settings is that of having a set routine for sleeping for everybody. Not so long ago, it was common practice to start the getting ready for bed routine late in the afternoon so that everybody would be in bed by 6 or 7 o'clock.

In order to deliver person-centred care, each individual's usual pattern needs to be known. This is important for two reasons. First, if the pattern changes this can be looked into; it may be because the person is worried, in pain, cold at night, unwell, depressed or needs a review of their medication. Second, it is important to prevent a 'normal' sleep pattern from being interpreted as challenging behaviour. It is not uncommon for older people to get up in the night, or to need one or more naps in the day. If it is usual for a person to get up in the night, this needs to be recorded so that the care plan can spell out what that person needs when they get up at night. This will undoubtedly vary from person to person; for example, one person may need to have the light turned on, to sip a warm drink and chat for a little while; another may need to physically get up and walk around; another may be awake and agitated because he is confused about what time it is and where he is – he will need reassurance and gentle reorientating. Similarly, for a person who naps in the day it may be far more comfortable and refreshing for them to be offered the opportunity to lie down for these naps rather than fall asleep in a chair and this too needs to be recorded.

In long-term care settings, the old culture of care has tended towards fairly fixed bedtime/wake time expectations for elderly residents with little flexibility for individuals. This has resulted in poor care practice where carers are likely to view wakefulness at night as a challenging behaviour which in turn has led to the widespread use of medication to reduce wakefulness at night. While some medication for some people can be very effective (Alzheimer's Society 2008), it is considered good practice in dementia care to look for alternatives in the first instance for the following reasons:

- Sleeping tablets lose their effect quite quickly, so you have to take more and more to get the same effect.

- They don't work for very long.

- Sleeping tablets can leave you tired and irritable the next day.

- Excessive sedation at bedtime may make the person unable to wake to go to the toilet and incontinence may occur.

- If they do wake, despite sedation, increased confusion and unsteadiness may occur.

- Tolerance develops quickly, and dependency can follow.

- Some people become addicted to them. The longer you take sleeping tablets, the more likely you are to become physically or psychologically dependent on them.

- These drugs are best used intermittently rather than regularly and should be reviewed regularly by the GP.

- If they are needed, they should not be used for longer than two weeks. (Royal College of Psychiatrists 2008)

In person-centred care, the emphasis is on supporting individualised sleeping routines while at the same time being able to judge and help when a particular sleep pattern for a particular individual is contributing to poor health or a state of ill-being.

Use the profile column to record as much as you know of the person's individual sleeping pattern during the day and during the night. For example 'Yvette rarely sleeps during the day; she retires to bed between 10.00 pm and

12.00 am and regularly gets up once or twice in the night. Yvette usually sleeps until 8.30 or 9.00 am in the morning.' 'Peter has several short naps in the day, usually after meals and sleeps soundly from 8.00 pm until 4.00 am after which time he tends to get up and potter.'

The special needs column is where to record what the person needs in order to comfortably maintain their own pattern. For example, in this column you might write 'Yvette likes company at bedtime to have a brief chat, enjoy a warm drink and say goodnight. Yvette needs to wear bed socks to keep her feet warm at night, even in the summer. When she wakes in the night, she needs reminding that it is night time, to be reassured that all her family are well, that they know where she is and that they will be visiting soon. Sometimes she likes another warm drink before being helped back to bed.' 'Peter goes to bed independently and likes to be left to potter in his room when he wakes at around 4.00 am before having another doze at 6.00 am.'

If the person you are profiling reports any difficulties with sleeping, or you observe that the person is uncomfortable during sleeping, avoiding sleeping or sleeping too much, you may need to consider a more detailed assessment in which case you should tick the specialist assessment box and write this up as a care need.

Sleeping difficulties might be related to emotional problems:

- anxiety and worry

- depression – which can cause very early morning waking and difficulty getting back to sleep

- thinking over and over about day-to-day problems

- missing a partner or another important attachment figure such as a pet or a cuddly toy.

Or there may be physical or practical reasons for sleeping difficulties:

- illness, pain or a high temperature

- apnoea – when breathing stops, due to throat tissue obstructing the airway and/or when the brain fails to control breathing during sleeping for more than twenty seconds

- not getting enough exercise

- eating too much which can make it difficult to get off to sleep

- going to bed hungry which can make you wake too early

- cigarettes, alcohol and drinks containing caffeine, such as tea and coffee

- the bedroom may be too noisy, too hot or too cold

- the bed may be uncomfortable or too small.

You and the person you are profiling and/or a friend or family member may be able to look at these areas and explore whether they are affecting healthy sleep. One of the advantages of enriched care planning is that you will be able to use information you gain about all areas of the person's life, such as life story and lifestyle to enrich your understanding of problems relating to sleep and other health issues.

If you and the person you are profiling feel that help from a specialist is a good idea you should seek consent from the person you are profiling and then involve the person's GP or approach a specialist nurse, occupational therapist, physiotherapist or your nearest sleep clinic.

On page three of the Health Template there is space to write down important information about the condition of the person's eyes, ears, teeth and gums, heart and lungs, feet and skin. There is also space to record relevent information about specific health issues to do with gender in the Women's/Men's Health Issues section. Finally at the bottom of this page, there is space for recording information about pain and about any identified risks to the person's overall health and well being.

Eyes and vision

It goes without saying that keeping our eyes healthy so that we can see well is important for all of us and arguably even more important for a person who has dementia. This is mainly because poor eyesight might exacerbate confusion and disorientation. Most people who live with dementia are also going through the process of ageing which brings changes that, for some, weaken the eyes. This in turn can make it more difficult to see and it is not unusual for an older person to need to wear glasses to be able to see well. Having weak eyes is not in itself life-threatening but can be immensely disabling as well as posing health and safety risks for example falling, bumping into things, or sustaining other injuries such as cuts and burns. This is one of the reasons why it is so important for *anybody* over the age of seventy to have an eye examination, which should be free of charge and carried out by a properly qualified optometrist or optician once a year. The optician will have the right techniques and equipment to assess sight and the health of the eyes generally, even for a person with severe dementia, and arrange for the right glasses or other treatment to be provided.

The optician will also detect and give advice about a range of common eye conditions which might include:

- **Glaucoma** caused by too much fluid pressure inside the eye leading to loss of vision and, if left untreated, blindness.

- **Cataracts** which are cloudy areas in the eye's lens causing loss of eyesight.

- **Retinal disorders** which damage the retina – a thin tissue that lines the back of the eye and sends light signals to the brain. Ageing and diabetes increase the risk of retinal disorder.

- **Corneal diseases and conditions** which can cause redness, watery eyes, pain, lower vision, or a halo effect. The cornea is the clear, dome-shaped 'window' at the front of the eye.

- **Floaters** which are tiny specks or 'cobwebs' that seem to float across the eyes usually in well-lit rooms or outdoors on a bright day. Floaters can be a normal part of ageing although sometimes they are a sign of a more serious eye problem, such as retinal detachment.

- **Tearing** (or having too many tears) can come from being sensitive to light, wind or temperature changes. Protecting your eyes, by wearing sunglasses for example, may solve the problem. Sometimes, tearing may mean a more serious eye problem, such as an infection or a blocked tear duct.

- **Dry eye** caused when tear glands don't work well causing itching, burning or vision loss.

- **Eyelid problems** can come from different diseases or conditions. Common eyelid problems include red and swollen eyelids, itching, tearing, being sensitive to light, and crusting of eyelashes during sleep.

Visual difficulties caused by poor eyesight and these other conditions can be managed well under the care of a good optician.

However, there may be other reasons why a person who has dementia is experiencing visual difficulties, namely, because of damage to the cortex of their brain. The cortex processes the images brought to it by the eyes. So, while poor eyesight can be helped by glasses, poor visual processing cannot. So, the first thing to ask at this point in the health profile is when the person last had an eye test. You may need to look elsewhere to get this information, for example in old case notes, or you may need to contact family members or previous carers to find this out. There is a space for writing this date on the template. If you are unsuccessful and you and the person you are profiling simply don't know, you write 'not known' by the date and then tick the 'I would like a specialist assessment' box and arrange for an eye test as soon as possible.

If the person you are caring for has had a recent eye check, and is doing everything that has been recommended by the optician, for example wearing glasses, but is still having visual difficulties, you may be able to explore this further when you come to use the Cognitive Ability Template.

In the 'Eyes and Vision' section, use the profile column to write down all the information you collect in relation to the person's eyes, eyelids and eyesight. You include here what the person with dementia says about their eyes but you may also need to discuss any observations that you have made and write these down too as well as checking to find out any previous medical history in relation to their eyes. For example 'Yvette had surgery for cataracts six months ago and has recovered well. She is short sighted and prone to headaches if she is in bright daylight or sunshine.' If the person uses anything to help their eyes such as glasses or eye drops these should be recorded in the special needs column. 'Yvette wears glasses for reading and needs reminding to find them and wear them. She must wear sunglasses when she is outdoors.'

If the person has not had an eye check in the last year, or they are experiencing any unpleasant or unusual visual experiences, discomfort or pain in their eyes or their eyelids, or they report recent increased difficulty with seeing things, you should record this also in the profile column, tick the 'specialist assessment' box and arrange for an eye test as soon as possible. Any immediate action like this that you need to take as a result of profiling the person's health should also be written up in the care plan.

Ears and hearing

The reason it is so important to ensure that the person's ears are healthy, and that their hearing is at its optimum, is because ear problems can be very uncomfortable and poor hearing makes it difficult to communicate. Lack or loss of communication brought on by deafness will put any person who also has dementia at risk of physical and social isolation. They are also at greater risk of accidents because they may not hear warning alarms and sirens. It has been so easy in the old culture of care to overlook and under-estimate the additional disability brought about by hearing difficulty. In this day and age, you may still come across the 'old culture' attitude that poor communication is part of getting older and not worth bothering about for people who are confused and disorientated anyway. In good person-centred care, the person is valued as a citizen with just as much right to a hearing test and treatment as anybody else. The ability to communicate is an essential part of living in human society. Advances in technology have led to an explosion of devices, gadgets and other methods to help people with hearing loss listen to and talk to others.

The most common cause of hearing loss is ageing and three quarters of people who are deaf are over sixty. Yet, research into this area finds that despite hearing loss being so common, the provision of hearing aids is inadequate among elderly people in the UK. Furthermore, and somewhat depressingly, the research found that socially disabling hearing loss is common even when hearing aids are used (Smeeth *et al.* 2001).

There are different levels of deafness. These are mild, moderate, severe or profound. People with mild deafness may have to work very hard to follow what is being said to them especially in noisy situations. People with moderate deafness would most likely need a hearing aid to follow what is being said to them. A person assessed to be severely deaf is likely to rely a lot on lip-reading, even with a hearing aid. British Sign Language (BSL) may be their first or preferred language. Profoundly deaf people understand speech by lip-reading. BSL may be their first or preferred language.

A healthy hearing system needs clean healthy ears because the external parts of our ear act like a trumpet to collect sound. Inside the ear is an organ known as the cochlea; this needs to be in good working order too because it is responsible for converting the mechanical vibration of sound into electrical signals. These can then be detected by the brain.

Hearing loss is caused when any part of the hearing system is blocked or damaged. Causes can range from wax blocking the ear canal and age-related changes to the sensory cells of the cochlea to brain damage. Given the high likelihood of an older person having some hearing loss, and the added difficulty that a person who has dementia might have reporting this, it is good practice to recommend an annual hearing check. There is a space in the Health Template to record the date of the last known hearing test; if the date is not known you should, with consent from the person, tick the 'specialist assessment' box and arrange for one.

As we get older, we naturally begin to find that our hearing gets worse, because the nerves that carry sounds from the ears to the brain die and are not replaced. Hearing loss in old age is usually gradual, and often begins with being unable to hear the most high-pitched sounds. A qualified audiologist will be able to test for normal hearing and recommend the right type of hearing aid to compensate if hearing loss is detected.

Other tests may be needed to find out the cause and this would need to start with a GP who will do a physical examination of the outside of the ear and possibly refer on to a specialist for further tests in the Ear, Nose and Throat (ENT) department of the hospital.

The most common causes of deafness include:

- **Ear wax** which is a yellowish waxy substance secreted in the ear canal. It is very important for cleaning and lubricating the ear as well as giving protection against bacteria, fungi and insects. However, if too much ear wax builds up and becomes impacted in the ear this can cause hearing loss.

- **Ear infections** can occur at any age and are caused when the middle ear space becomes filled with mucus (fluid), often during a cold. The mucus may then become infected by bacteria or viruses. The main symptoms are earache and feeling unwell.

- **Glue ear**, a condition which causes fluid to build up in the middle ear. This is a common childhood problem but can occur at any age.

- **Foreign body obstruction** which means any object that is in the ear lobe or ear canal, that is not meant to be there and could cause harm without immediate medical attention. Objects usually found in the ear lobe are earrings, either stuck in the lobe from infection or placed too deep during insertion. Foreign bodies that might find their way into a person's ear canal can include food, insects, and ordinary small objects such as buttons, beads, pieces of cloth or tissue.

- **Presbyacusis** is the medical term for the hearing loss of older people and is caused by the degeneration of nerve cells in the ear. The hearing loss comes on gradually, often over several years.

- **Side effects of medication** can include hearing loss which can usually be reversed once the medication is stopped. The symptoms include a noise or ringing sensation in the ear, a pressure in the ear, and a spinning sensation that may or may not have nausea as a side effect. If hearing loss comes on while taking a medication this may be a sign that the medication is causing some hearing loss. Drugs that might cause hearing loss as a side effect include aspirin and products containing aspirin, nonsteroidal anti inflammatory drugs and some antibiotics if given intravenously.

- **Acoustic neuroma** is a rare, non-cancerous brain tumour which grows on the acoustic nerve and affects hearing and balance. Hearing is normally predominantly affected in one ear. Symptoms include ringing in the ear, dizziness, facial numbness, tingling or pain, headaches, temporary sight problems and earache.

- **Ménière's disease**, a rare progressive disorder which causes fluid to build up in the inner ear disrupting both balance and hearing. Symptoms include attacks of vertigo which brings dizziness, nausea, vomiting, palpitations and sweating; tinnitus which causes sounds in your ear or head; and hearing loss.

If a hearing test shows that a person does not have normal hearing, other tests can be carried out to find out the cause. Their doctor may do a physical examination of the outside of the ear. They might be referred to a specialist for further tests, in the Ear, Nose and Throat (ENT) department of a hospital. Hearing difficulties caused by these conditions can be managed well under the care of a good practice nurse or GP.

However, there may be other reasons why a person who has dementia is experiencing hearing difficulties, namely, because of damage to the cortex of their brain. The cortex processes the sounds brought to it by the ears. So, while poor hearing might be helped by a hearing aid, poor visual processing cannot, Chapter 6 deals with this. So, the first thing to ask at this point in the health profile is when the person last had a hearing test. You may need to look elsewhere to get this information, for example in old case notes, or you may need to contact family members or previous carers to find this out. There is a space for writing this date on the template. If you are unsuccessful and you and the person you are profiling simply don't know, you write 'not known' by the date and then tick the 'I would like a specialist assessment' box and arrange for a hearing test as soon as possible.

If the person you are caring for has had a recent hearing check, and is doing everything that has been recommended by the audiologist and the other professionals involved, for example wearing a hearing aid, but is still having hearing difficulties, you may be able to explore this further when you come to use the Cognitive Ability Template.

In the 'Ears and Hearing' section, use the profile column to write down all the information you collect in relation to the person's ears and their hearing. You should include here what the person with dementia says about this but you may also need to discuss any observations that you have made and write these down too as well as checking to find out any previous medical history in relation to their ears and hearing. For example 'James had treatment for an ear infection three months ago and has recovered well. He is hard of hearing especially in his left ear. He is also prone to wax build-up in both ears.'

If the person has been prescribed or uses anything to help their ears such as a hearing aid these should be recorded in the special needs column. 'James has got a hearing aid but he doesn't like wearing it. He needs to be encouraged and reminded to wear it; and he needs people around him to speak into his right ear.' If you and James think it would be a good idea to learn about more specialised communication aids and techniques, you should tick the 'I would like a specialist assessment' box and make a referral to a speech and language therapist or an occupational therapist.

If the person has not had a hearing check in the last year, you should make a referral to a local audiologist. Or if they are experiencing any unpleasant or unusual auditory experiences, ringing or buzzing in the ear, dizziness or loss of balance, ear pain that is severe or goes on for more than twenty-four hours or fluid or blood coming out of the ear, you should refer them to their GP.

Teeth and gums

Good oral health has a very positive impact on well-being with benefits not only for general health but also for dignity and self-esteem, social integration and general nutrition (Fiske *et al.* 2006). Poor oral health can lead to pain and tooth loss, and both make it difficult to enjoy life, to communicate and to eat. Gum disease is very common in adults and if left untreated can lead to tooth decay. The majority of people manage, with support from their dentist, to look after their gums and their teeth throughout their lives and to keep most if not all of their own teeth. People who have lost their teeth wear dentures; but they still need to keep their dentures clean and to look after their gums. A person who has dementia, whether they have their own teeth or whether they wear dentures, is likely to need help to maintain good oral health in order to avoid the pain and discomfort of gum disease, tooth decay and the consequent exacerbation of distress and confusion.

There are two main types of dental disease which it may be useful for you to know about:

- **Gum (periodontal) disease** which can lead to bleeding and inflamed gums. Other symptoms of gum disease include receding gums, loose teeth and bad breath. It is caused by a build-up of plaque which can be reduced greatly by regular cleaning.

- **Tooth decay (dental caries)** happens when the sugar from sugary foods sits on plaque to make acid which attacks the tooth. Again, regular cleaning to keep the plaque at bay and the avoidance of sugary foods reduce the risk of tooth decay.

If the person you are profiling would not be able to cope with a regular check-up from a local dentist, you can make a referral to your local salaried primary dental care service which might be called community or personal dental service. There should be a dentist available from within this service who can provide dental care for people with disabilities and complex medical conditions. Details of your local salaried dental service are obtainable from your local primary care trust.

In this section of the health profile, you record any current unmet dental needs that need immediate attention. You should ask the person you are profiling if they feel any pain or discomfort in their mouth. You may also need to observe the person over a period of time. Possible signs of underlying dental problems include:

- refusal to eat (particularly hard or cold foods)

- frequent pulling at the face or mouth

- leaving previously worn dentures out of the mouth

- increased restlessness, moaning or shouting

- disturbed sleep

- refusal to take part in daily activities

- aggressive behaviour.

If the person tells you that they are experiencing pain or discomfort in their mouth, or shows any of the above signs, it may be that a referral needs to be made to a dentist. Record what has been said or what you have observed in the profile column. For example 'James says his tooth hurts and he has been off his food lately'. Also tick the specialist assessment box and then, in the first instance, you could arrange with consent from the person for a nurse to take a look and decide what course of action to take.

It will be helpful to find out anyway when the person last had a dental check. There is a space for writing this date on the template. If you are unsuccessful and you and the person you are profiling simply don't know, you write 'not known' by the date and then tick the 'I would like a specialist assessment' box and arrange for a dental check as soon as possible.

If the person you are caring for has had a recent dental check, you should record this too in the profile column detailing special needs such as dentures and mouthwashes in the special needs column. Use the profile column to write down all the information you collect in relation to the how the person currently looks after their teeth and gums and the special needs column to record the help they currently receive to do so. For example, you might write 'James cleans his teeth once a day after breakfast' in the profile column and 'he needs to have the toothpaste on the toothbrush presented to him and a little verbal encouragement' in the special needs column.

Any current special needs, along with any other immediate action that you need to take as a result of profiling the person's teeth and gums should also be written up in their Enriched Care Plan.

Heart and lungs

The risk of developing heart or lung conditions increases with age and the person you are profiling may need your help to manage an existing condition or to recognise and deal with a new or developing condition. Use this section of the Health Template to explore both. Breathing problems and poor circulation may be signs of underlying heart or lung conditions.

Breathing problems

Common breathing problems include shortness of breath, chest discomfort, wheezing and coughing. These can be experienced at any age and although they are common, they should not be overlooked as a normal part of ageing. There may be an underlying medical condition such as pneumonia, angina, coronary heart disease and heart failure, a neurological disorder (such as stroke), or cancer. Breathing problems are also sometimes linked to sinus problems, colds, anaemia, asthma and allergies. Carrying excess body weight may also make a person more prone to breathing problems.

A person who has dementia may need your help

- to notice and report breathing problems to the doctor

- to make sure that any current treatment routine for breathing problems is followed and that medicines are taken properly.

In this part of the Health Profile you should record any newly observed or reported discomfort or difficulties the person has with their breathing as well as known conditions that require treatment. Newly observed or reported problems would include sudden chest pain or tightness during exercise or walking or at rest; neck pain; pain in the throat or arms; a choking feeling; laboured, rapid or shallow breathing or shortness of breath. You should seek medical advice immediately for any of these. Other changes to look out for include persistent coughing. If the person is coughing up blood or the colour of their phlegm changes or if they become short of breath during activities such as walking you should also seek medical advice.

Known conditions and current treatments should be recorded here too. These are conditions that have been medically diagnosed, and require ongoing treatment such as chronic obstructive pulmonary disease (COPD), pulmonary emphysema, chronic bronchitis and asthma. Treatments for these may require the use of an oxygen cylinder, nebuliser or bronchodilator which is a small spray can containing medicine that acts directly on the person's air passages and/or oral medicines which are swallowed. It is very important that the instructions for using or taking these are followed properly. If the person you are profiling needs your help and you are not sure about the proper way to help them to use the equipment or to take these medicines you should ask a trained nurse or a doctor to teach you.

Poor circulation

The risk of developing poor circulation of the blood around the body increases with age and can be caused by serious underlying medical conditions. Poor circulation, if left untreated, can also cause damage to vital organs, limbs and peripheral body parts such as toes and fingers. The person you are profiling may have pre-existing poor circulation or they may develop poor circulation and you can play an important role in recognising and reporting potential problems.

Signs of poor circulation include:

- cold hands and feet

- white fingers

- tenderness of body parts

- bluish discoloration of body parts

- pain, soreness when walking

- accumulation of fluid under the skin of the hands, arms, feet, ankles, legs (oedema)

- dizziness when standing quickly

- numbness of body parts

- migraine headaches

- tinnitus and hearing loss.

Some people with reduced circulation complain of cold hands and feet. If you observe that the person's feet or tips of their fingers are pale in colour or even slightly blue tinged then this may indicate an underlying circulatory problem. If any of these symptoms are observed or reported during the health profiling process you should seek medical advice so that serious illness can be ruled out or treated and further health issues prevented.

Having breathing or circulatory problems can be very frightening for the person and may impact on the person's ability to engage fully in activities. Profiling the nature of the problems will help you better identify the needs and abilities of the person so that you can tailor your care accordingly.

You should record any known or observed breathing or circulation problems or conditions in the profile column of the 'Heart and Lungs' section. For example 'Yvette becomes short of breath when she walks for any length of time. We believe this is due to her asthma which was diagnosed by her GP two years ago. However, she also has a persistent cough and this is new.' In the special needs column you would record information about what the person needs in order to manage their condition and keep safe and well. For example 'Yvette needs to avoid dusty rooms and contact with cats; she also uses her bronchodilator independently. She needs help to ensure that this is with her, in her handbag at all times.'

Any breathing or circulation problems that have not been medically assessed warrant a referral to the GP and you should tick the specialist assessment box. In this example, you would tick the box because Yvette's cough is something new and needs to be assessed by her GP. Such a need would be carried forward as part of the person's Enriched Care Plan and dealt with as soon as possible as a matter of urgency.

Feet

Healthy feet are essential for keeping active, mobile and engaged with the world and this may be especially important for a person who has dementia. Foot problems can be inherited or can develop as a side effect of other illnesses such as diabetes and rheumatoid arthritis or can appear in middle age from wearing ill-fitting shoes (The Disability Foundation 2006).

In this section, you need to find out and record any foot problems that have not been sorted out, foot problems that have been previously managed and how these are managed, and what the person does and needs to keep their feet healthy. As with profiling ears, eyes, teeth and gums, an initial step is to find out if the person is experiencing any pain or discomfort. Some people who have dementia find it difficult to talk about, remember and/or locate pain and so it is always a good idea to focus on the here and now. Unlike ears, eyes, teeth and gums, feet are easy to look at.

Ask the person to look at their feet and, if appropriate, take off socks and shoes and then talk about how their feet feel. Together, you can assess:

- whether shoes, socks, stockings, tights, slippers are comfortable and well-fitting; it is useful to include the size of the person's foot in this section

- that both feet are clean and dry

- that toenails are not too long or ingrown or infected

- whether there are any corns or other growths or marks that need assessing

- whether there is any swelling, pain or skin discoloration.

You should record how the person's feet look and feel in the profile column and tick the specialist assessment box if you think there may be a problem. If the person has already had an assessment, either by a GP or a chiropodist, you should record this too. Then, in the special needs column write any treatment or special help that the person currently has to keep their feet healthy.

Many older people at home and in long-term care settings benefit from regularly seeing a chiropodist who is a specialist trained to inspect, detect and treat foot conditions and to provide foot care education. Any person who, for any reason, cannot look after their own feet, or who has rheumatoid arthritis, mobility or sight problems or who cannot reach or see their own feet should be referred to a chiropodist.

Common problems that can be helped include: corns, calluses, verrucas (warts caused by a virus), athlete's foot (easily spread fungal infection treated with anti-fungal cream or powder), hard skin, nail and skin conditions, toenail cutting, ingrowing toenails (Society of Chiropodists and Podiatrists 2008).

Skin

A person who has dementia is at greater risk of developing a skin condition if they are also elderly, under-active, dehydrated, bed or chair bound or poorly nourished. Poor skin can be very uncomfortable, even painful, and furthermore can lead to or be a sign of a more serious health condition.

In this part of the profiling process, you need to find out whether the person you are profiling has any unmet needs in relation to their skin and also what their current routine is for keeping their skin healthy including any special treatments or therapies that they need. So, the first question is likely to be about the condition of the person's skin at the moment. You should talk directly to the person about this but you may also need to look at the person's skin with them, or arrange for somebody appropriate, such as a nurse or doctor to do so. Previous episodes of skin conditions are relevant to know about too. The person may be able to tell you about this, but, if not, you should ask their permission to find out from their family or from their medical records.

Skin conditions in older people include the following.

Moles

Some moles are present at birth, some develop during adolescence and adulthood and some are common in older people who have spent a lot of time in the sun. The old age moles or seborrhoeic keratoses are raised, quite faint at the edge and can vary in colour. Most moles are normal and harmless, but in a few cases they can develop skin cancer and so should be checked routinely to make sure that they do not change size or shape or begin to bleed, ooze or become red or itchy.

Pigment changes

These are brown spots or freckles which are usually harmless. They only become a cause for concern if they become thicker and bigger or develop a crust.

Purpura

Changes in an older person's skin and blood vessels can result in bruising which is referred to as senile purpura and usually affects the arms. These bruises can take longer to heal but are no cause for concern.

Scabies

Scabies can be a concern in group living situations because it is infectious. Scabies is an infestation of microscopic mites in the skin; and any person with dry or cracked skin is more at risk of becoming infested. It causes intense itching, especially at night, and looks like a pimply rash. The rash is more likely to develop within skin folds and on the wrist, elbow, knee, penis, breast, or shoulder blades. If left untreated, the person can scratch so much that sores develop and these can become infected.

Leg ulcers

Leg ulcers can happen to older people who have high blood pressure and poor circulation. The ulcers make the legs swell up and either become pale or turn a reddish-brown colour. The condition can be extremely painful and cause reduced mobility and sleep disturbance which, in turn, can cause a reduction in energy levels.

Pressure ulcers (bed sores)

People who are bed or chair bound are most likely to have bed sores which erupt because of unrelieved pressure to the skin. These days, there are excellent preventative and symptom relief therapies and equipment available to greatly reduce the risk of bed sores.

Use the profile column to write any information that you collect either through talking or observation. For example 'Yvette has some moles on her body that have been there for many years and are not a cause for concern. She also has dry skin on her legs.' In the special needs column, you should make a note of any creams or tablets or special equipment that the person currently uses. 'Yvette has a bath once a week and uses a moisturising bath foam; she also needs reminding to rub barrier cream into her legs every night.'

If the person reports or shows any discomfort or pain or there are changes in how their skin looks, you should, with their permission, tick the specialist assessment box and arrange for a district nurse or a GP to undertake a skin assessment.

Women's and men's health issues

There are some health risks and conditions that are specific to being female or male. These can occur at any time in a man or a woman's adult life, including later years. The person you are profiling may have one or more known conditions which still need to be managed, or which develop as something new alongside living with dementia. This part of the health profile is to help you to help the person you are profiling to manage existing conditions, reduce the risk of these reoccurring and to notice symptoms that need to be checked out.

The most common women's health conditions include:

- breast cancer

- ovarian, vulval or womb cancer

- endometriosis

- pelvic inflammatory disease

- pelvic prolapse.

The most common men's health conditions include:

- prostate cancer

- prostatism

- testicular cancer

- male thrush.

Women

All women between the ages of fifty and seventy years of age should be invited for regular screening checks to pick up early signs of breast cancer. Women over seventy must make their own appointment. You may need to help the woman you are profiling to find out when she last had a mammogram and whether or not she is due for another one. If she is due or if she doesn't know you can tick the 'I require a specialist assessment' box and, with her consent, help her to arrange this.

Women who have been sexually active in their lives and who are between the ages of forty-nine and sixty-five should have a cervical smear test every five years. Women over sixty-four can stop having smear tests if the previous two in the past ten years have been negative. The person you are profiling may need your help to find out whether or not she needs and wants a cervical smear. Tick the specialist assessment box if she wishes you to go ahead and help her to arrange a smear.

Ovarian cancer often presents few or no symptoms. The most important factor is whether it is in the family. As part of the health profiling process, you may need to help her to find out whether she or any of her family has any previous history of ovarian cancer. If the answer is 'yes' she is probably entitled to an ovarian screening and a doctor's appointment needs to be arranged. In this case you should write the history in the profile column and tick the specialist assessment box.

Vulval cancer is relatively rare but the risk increases in women over fifty years. If the person you are profiling experiences

- pain or burning during urination

- bleeding or discharge

- discomfort, pain, itching or burning of the vulva

- lumps on the skin

you should tick the specialist assessment box and help her to get medical attention as soon as possible.

The most common symptom of womb cancer is abnormal vaginal bleeding. In more advanced stages of the disease, tiredness, nausea, loss of appetite, weight loss, constipation or pain in the back or legs may occur.

Endometriosis is not a condition that presents after the menopause. However, if the person has had treatment for this condition in the past, she may be more at risk of developing osteoporosis which may be of relevance now.

Prolapse of the pelvic organs happens more commonly in older women and is caused when the supporting muscles in the pelvis become too weak to hold in the organs of the pelvis such as the womb (uterus) or bladder. Symptoms may include:

- heaviness or pressure in the pelvis

- a bulge of tissue in the genital area, which can be quite alarming, and is often red and sore

- urinary problems and loss of bladder control

- pain in the pelvis or lower back

- constipation

- vaginal discharge or bleeding.

If any of these conditions are currently being treated or have been treated in the past, you should write this down in the profile column. For example 'Yvette suffered from endometriosis as a young woman and had a hysterectomy twenty-six years ago. There is a history of ovarian cancer in her family. Yvette is seventy-one but she has not had a mammogram or any screening tests in the last seven years.'

In the special needs column you should write down any measures that are being taken or that need to be taken to keep Yvette well and healthy in relation to women's health issues: 'Yvette takes vitamin D supplements daily to boost her bones. She is overdue for a mammogram and needs to be assessed by a doctor for screening of ovarian cancer which is in her family.' You would tick the specialist assessment box and, with her consent, arrange for these as soon as possible.

Men

The most common cancer in men is prostate cancer and the risk becomes higher in the over-fifty age group. Causes are not clear but are believed to be related to high fat/meat with low vegetable diet. The risk increases for men who have a history of it in the family and ethnic origin seems to be a factor too with Asian men being more at risk than Afro-Caribbean or African-American men. Treatment is usually very successful if diagnosis is made early.

There may be no symptoms but, if there are, these would include:

- difficulty or delay passing urine

- urinating more often than usual

- a weak stream

- stopping and starting

- feeling the bladder isn't empty and continually needing to go to the toilet

- dribbling after passing urine

- pain while urinating

- blood in the urine

- pain or stiffness in the lower back, pelvis and hips.

When men reach age forty years, their prostate gland starts to get bigger. For some this does not cause a problem, but for others, it does. Prostatism (enlarged prostate gland) may cause some or all of these symptoms:

- difficulty passing urine

- a weak irregular stream

- dribbling after passing urine

- feeling the bladder isn't empty

- feeling the need to go to the toilet continuously

- having to get up throughout the night to pass water

- having to find a loo urgently when out and about.

Taking antibiotics, having diabetes and/or low immune levels all increase the risk of male thrush. This condition is usually managed by using an anti-fungal cream (clotrimazole) along with good hygiene.

The symptoms include:

- inflammation, redness, soreness, appearance of spots or itching at the head of the penis

- build-up of secretions under the foreskin.

In the profile column, write down any known issues that currently require managing. For example 'James was diagnosed with prostatism three years ago.' In the special needs column, record what James needs to do to manage his condition. 'James manages this condition by avoiding alcohol and caffeine and eating a low fat diet and plenty of red tomatoes. He needs help to keep up his outpatients appointments so that this condition can be monitored.'

You should also record any observed or reported problems which might be new in the profile column. These would include any of the symptoms listed above, but also any lumps, spots, rashes, swelling, discharge, pain or discomfort warrants a referral to the doctor. For example 'James has a rash around his groin area and he says it is uncomfortable and itchy.' Here, you would tick the specialist assessment box and, with his consent, make an appointment for James to see the doctor.

If any of these symptoms are reported or observed you should tick the specialist assessment box and seek medical advice as soon as possible.

Pain

It is still a common misconception that people who have dementia cannot feel pain. The fact is that dementia does not alter the fundamental experience of pain (Personal Social Services Research Unit 2005). It is true that dementia can affect a person's ability to remember that they have been in pain or to report that they are in pain. For this reason, it is very important for carers to be on the look out for any signs of pain. Of course, many people living with dementia can and do report pain when they experience it, and may need other kinds of help managing their pain.

The 'Pain' section of the profiling template is for recording any unmet needs in relation to pain and any current recognised pain along with information about how the person manages this and the help they need. You may prefer to use a more detailed pain assessment instead of or in conjunction with this. The Abbey Pain Scale (Abbey 2007) has been developed specifically for use with people who have dementia. There is also an excellent Pain in Dementia Fact Sheet developed by the Personal Social Services Research Unit available on the internet which provides information for carers about helping people who have dementia to manage pain. Contact details are included in the list of useful resources at the back of this book.

Asking about and looking out for signs of pain should be a continuous process and family members and carers are in the best position to be able to do this naturally as they help the person through their ordinary day-to-day activities. The risk of pain for a person who has dementia is extremely high. Causes are often down to untreated underlying physical conditions. These are numerous but include

- urinary tract infections

- fractures

- sore or infected mouth

- skin or eye conditions

- arthritis

- constipation.

When you discuss pain with the person you are profiling and using words to communicate is difficult, it can be a good idea to start with the question 'Have you got any pain anywhere?' but then to go through each part of the body starting with the feet. Ask the person to look at their feet and then ask if their feet are comfortable or not. Move up the body and ask about legs, stomach, private parts, chest, shoulders, arms, back, neck, head. If appropriate you can lightly touch or pat the body part you are discussing or even use pictures or a doll. This may help the person you are profiling to focus. Try and stick with simple 'yes/no' questions and use other words such as 'sore', 'hurting', 'aching' or 'uncomfortable' as well as the word 'pain'. This will make it much easier for the person to really understand what you are asking about.

You may need to rely on observation as a way of finding out if the person you are profiling is experiencing pain. There are a number of ways this might be communicated:

- **Behaviour:** unusual or changed behaviour such as fidgeting, restlessness, rocking, patting and other repetitive behaviour is often seen as part of the dementing process but can be a sign that the person is in pain. Also, holding the part of the body that hurts or curling up can indicate pain.

- **Mood:** untreated pain can cause a person to become depressed, withdrawn or tense and anxious.

- **Facial expression:** pain may cause frowning and grimacing.

- **Verbalising:** calling out, shouting, swearing and groaning are all natural responses to being in pain.

If in the course of discussion or observation, you have any concerns that the person may be in pain, you should write what has been said or what you have seen in the profile column, tick the specialised assessment box and arrange, with their consent, for the person to be physically examined by a nurse or a doctor. This of course will also have to be added to the person's Enriched Care Plan as a need.

Any current, known issues regarding pain should also be recorded in the profile column e.g. 'James suffers from headaches, he rubs his head repetitively when he has a headache.' Use the special needs column to record the help the person has to manage the pain: 'James has two x 200 mg paracetamol every two hours for the rest of the day when he has a headache. These need to be given to him with a glass of water and an explanation that they are tablets to make his headache go away.'

Helping a person who has dementia to recognise and manage pain is an ongoing and important part of the caring role which can do a lot to improve and maintain well-being.

Health and well-being risks

There is a space at the bottom of Page 3 for writing down any risks that come to light during the health profiling process. This is not in itself a formal risk assessment, just a quick and practical way of recording obvious risks so that they are known about within the care setting. You should record here what the person with dementia says about any risks that they feel are specific to them. For example, risk of falling or choking or getting lost. It might also be helpful to discuss any observations that you have made and write these down. If the person needs any special measures to be taken to reduce risks to their health and well-being such as good lighting at night to reduce the risk of falling, or mashed food to reduce the risk of choking, these should be recorded in the middle column. If the person has had a previous risk assessment, write this in the box and state where it is kept. If you think the person needs or might benefit from a risk assessment now, you can tick the specialist assessment box on the far right hand side and write it as a need in the Enriched Care Plan. Don't forget to include any mental health and well-being risks that come to light (see Page 4 of the Health Template). These might include risk of depression or anxiety or other upsetting feelings under certain circumstances. For example 'James is at risk of becoming angry and upset if he is with too many people at once or if too many people are speaking at once or if he is put under pressure.' 'Yvette is at risk of low mood and tearfulness if she is separated for too long from Danny, her rabbit.'

Mental health and well-being

This section of the Health Profiling Template is there to encourage and help you to discuss mental well-being and the diagnosis of dementia and what this means for the person. If you believe that the person has suffered from mental illness in the past but is unable or unwilling to discuss it, you should ask for permission to ask a family member or friend on their behalf. The following questions will be useful for completing this page of the template.

Mental well-being – have you ever suffered from depression?

Use this opportunity to discuss with the person how they have coped in the past with loss and change. Words such as 'feeling low' might be easier for the person to relate to than medical terminology.

Mental well-being – have you ever suffered from anxiety?

At the same time, you can discuss with the person whether or not they are prone to feelings of anxiety. Words such as 'churning stomach' or 'feeling in a panic' or 'dry mouth, sweating, worried' might be easier for the person to relate to than medical terminology.

Mental well-being – have you ever suffered from other unpleasant feelings?

There may be other unpleasant experiences that the person who has dementia has had or is experiencing now. These might include feeling that other people are talking about them or trying to harm them or that they have heard voices or seen upsetting sights. This is an opportunity to understand, from their perspective, what these experiences are like and how they affect the person.

Further space is provided in this section for writing down any additional information that the person wants others to know about, including things that other people have said or done in the past that have been helpful.

Dementia – have you had a diagnosis of a particular type of dementia?

There may be a reluctance or difficulty for family, friends and professionals to speak directly to a person who has dementia about dementia. Many people who have dementia, if they have been in care for a long time, may have not been formally diagnosed whereas a younger person still living at home may have had a specific diagnosis. For each individual, the situation around diagnosis and open talking will be different. What seems important for person-centred care is to be as open and honest as possible and for the word 'dementia' to become less taboo.

If you feel comfortable using this part of the profile, it can be very empowering and supportive for the person who has dementia. Talking openly about dementia gives the message that this is manageable, it is something that can be handled, it is something that lots of people experience.

Using words such as 'poor memory' or 'slower thinking' may be more appropriate and lead to a helpful discussion about how the person is experiencing their cognitive changes. Finding out directly from the person how they wish their condition to be referred to is positive and respectful. Some people may wish their own specific diagnosis to be referred to, for example 'Alzheimer's disease', while others may prefer to be described as having 'memory problems' and some may not wish to be given a label at all.

Dementia – diagnosistic details

If the person has had a diagnosis and they are happy to have this information documented, there is a section on Page 4 for recording the date of diagnosis and details of who made the diagnosis. There is also a space for recording the person's own description of their symptoms and a description of how the person wishes their condition to be referred to by other people. If the person has had previous cognitive assessments, these can be noted here. If the person would like to be referred for a specialist assessment, this should be noted here too.

IDENTIFYING AND DOCUMENTING NEEDS FROM THE HEALTH PROFILE

Identifying needs

Much of the work involved in identifying health needs will have already been done during the profiling process. If you have ticked 'I would like a specialist assessment' anywhere on the profile, this needs to be carried forward and documented as a need in the Enriched Care Plan along with any current interventions that are being provided to support the person's health.

Documenting needs

Having identified what is important for the person, you will now need to reflect this in what you write in the three working templates:

- Brief Profile Sheet
- Key Information Sheet
- The Enriched Care Plan.

Brief Profile Sheet

There is a space in the fourth section of the Brief Profile Sheet recording for 'Key Health and Risk Issues'. There is only room to briefly summarize the very important things, and you will need to talk to the person and/or their family to decide what these are. It may be helpful here to imagine what a new carer would absolutely need to know to maintain the person's health and safety. Health conditions such as diabetes and risks such as falling would be appropriate to mention here.

Key Information Sheet

Use the 'People that I may wish to contact' section to fill in names of anybody who is involved in helping the person to maintain good health such as the name of their own optician, chiropodist and district nurse.

The other section of relevance in the Key Information Sheet is further down the page and entitled 'Important information that I want people involved in my care to know about'. Again, if anything has come up during profiling of health that the person feels is very important for others to know about, it can be recorded here. This might be in relation to medication or specific problems which are not immediately obvious but that need to be known about such as allergies, blood type, or where emergency equipment is kept such as nebulisers.

Or the information might be in relation to mental health or the person's diagnosis of dementia.

The Enriched Care Plan

The end product, the Enriched Care Plan, will be drawn from all the profiling that you do in relation to life story, lifestyle and future wishes, personality, health, capacity for doing, cognitive ability and life at the moment. There are just three columns in the plan. On the left hand side is the column entitled 'I need'. The middle column is headed 'My carers will'. The right hand column is for recording a date for review.

At this stage in the enriched care planning process, you only need write in the 'I need' column in relation to needs arising from health issues.

Drawing from the examples used at the in the 'Using the Health Profiling Template' section of this chapter, here are some examples of what you would record in this column:

I need

- to be given my medication three times each day

- to eat my food with a teaspoon

- drinks to be placed in my hand so that I can drink independently

- to be referred for a mobility assessment

- to be given my stick when I need to move around

- a raised toilet and grab rails to be able to use the toilet independently

- company at bedtime and help to put my bedsocks on to keep my feet warm

- to be given my reading glasses when I want to read

- my carer to load my toothbrush with toothpaste and hand me my toothbrush so that I can brush my teeth independently

- to be taken to my chiropody appointment monthly

- 400 mg paracetamol four hourly when I have a headache.

SUMMARY

- A person who has dementia may not be able to report on or adequately manage their own physical or mental health issues and the risk of treatable health problems being missed can be high.

- It is good practice to explore poor health as a potential cause of changed behaviour or of ill-being or distress and to give priority to this when you are planning or reviewing the person's care.

- The Health Profiling Template provides a structure for finding out in detail about current health issues and treatments; how the person copes with everyday basic daily living activities; any potential unmet physical or mental health needs, risks, pain and the person's preference for addressing dementia.

- The Enriched Care Plan is to help you to help the person you are profiling to manage existing conditions, reduce the risk of these getting worse or reoccurring and to notice newly occurring physical or mental health symptoms that need medical attention.

Chapter 6

Capacity for Doing

Generally speaking, mature human beings have the capacity to engage with other people, tasks and objects, making it possible to live in the world without difficulty. In adulthood we are in full control of our thinking and our physical abilities and can use both, in harmony, to achieve what we set out to do. For the person with dementia however this may not be the case; 'doing' can become difficult or even impossible but, it is never the case that any person (unless in a coma) is completely unable to engage with their world.

The purpose then of profiling capacity for doing is to ensure that the carer(s) of the person being profiled have a clear care plan that details all the support needed to facilitate meaningful and achievable engagement for the person being profiled. This is most important if we want the dementia care workforce to move away from task-orientated care where carers do 'to' or 'for' based on the assumption that people who have dementia can't do anything. Delivering person-centred care means providing and supporting an environment in which the person who has dementia is able to live out their drive to engage with the world. All human beings, unless in a coma, are able to engage with their world in some way or other. As importantly, all human beings have a drive to engage with their world and a need and a right to do so. The psychological need for occupation is a challenging but not impossible need for person-centred workforces to meet in person-centred care.

ENGAGEMENT

The term 'doing' in enriched care planning is meant in its widest sense and is closely linked to the term 'engagement'. Engagement is a broad term for all the things we do to connect with the world around us ranging from gazing at objects or people right through to the more complex types of doing such as driving a car or cooking a meal. People who have dementia seem to be particularly at risk of not 'doing' or disengagement for a number of reasons including:

- old culture thinking that people who have dementia can't do anything

- people pulling back, avoiding or ignoring the person who has dementia

- the person being overwhelmed by the world around them often by an overloaded or unfamiliar environment with too much happening at the same time causing the person to withdraw

- being placed in an 'empty' space such as a large community lounge where there is nothing and nobody within reach to connect with

- being expected to engage with people, tasks or objects that have no meaning for the person or are too difficult to tackle or understand.

In order to reduce the risk of disengagement, carers need to make it easy for the person to engage with people, tasks and objects as part of their day-to-day role. For example:

- Go the extra mile to make eye contact, physical contact (a pat on the shoulder), verbal contact (hello) and non-verbal contact (a wave or other connecting gesture)

- Make everyday and important objects appropriate, interesting and within visual and physical reach, for example, personal belongings such as handbag, book, remote control should be on a reachable coffee table.

- Create a visually inviting environment that triggers action, for example, a duster on the table, a broom against the wall.

Carers also need to be able to understand enough about the person's capacity for doing. It's no help leaving a broom if the person can't see it to pick it up; it's no good arranging a skittles game if the person can't play skittles.

UNDERSTANDING CAPACITY FOR DOING

From babyhood, we develop our ability to 'do' gradually and in a certain order. First of all, we develop the ability to pick up, or grasp things. Once we have mastered this, we learn to tell the difference between and use different objects. Next we learn to keep going with what we are doing which in turn makes it possible to operate with a goal in mind.

Here is an explanation of how we develop our capacity for doing using a bunch of keys as an example. When we are just a few weeks old, we can only gaze at the keys; if somebody jingles them we will also engage through listening. Looking and listening are both important sensory ways of engaging with the world. By the time we are crawling, we are also able to pick up the keys; we have learned to grasp objects. The next ability we develop is that of being able to do something with the object. By throwing the keys on the floor, we learn that there is more than just one object in the world – there are two. There are the keys and the floor. We are learning to understand difference and distinguish between objects. Through trial and error we learn to note the effects of our actions; if we drop the keys on the floor, they make a sound and cause people around us to react; and this makes it possible for us to develop the ability to use objects to achieve a goal. By the time we are walking and running around, we will be learning to use the keys to lock and unlock doors. This is goal-directed action. The journey from being only able to look at and listen to the keys to being able to use them proficiently to lock and unlock doors is made possible by human cognitive development. Cognitive means to do with thinking and all human beings need to develop physically as well as cognitively in order to able to 'do'.

An American occupational therapist, Claudia Kay Allen, used this understanding of how we develop as a basis for her 'Cognitive Disabilities Model'. This model is based on the idea that the skills for doing develop in the sequence described above (Allen Earhart and Blue 1992).

Here is a simplified summary of how our doing skills develop:

First skill: turn head to look at object

Second skill: grasp object

Third skill: use hands to manipulate objects

Fourth skill: begin to use simple tools

Fifth skill: note effects of actions

Sixth skill: sequence actions through known steps

Allen's model is based on the idea that we need the first skill before we can develop the second; we need the second skill before we can develop the third and so on. The same applies to physical skills, hence the familiar saying about not being able to run before one can walk.

The usefulness of this model for supporting a person who has dementia lies in understanding that losing a doing skill alters the person's comfortable mode of doing. So, for example if a person loses the skill of being able to note the effect of their action on objects, they will struggle to engage in goal-directed action; their comfortable mode of doing changes.

The model has a theoretical base and assessment tools used by occupational therapists to assess the mode of doing which is easiest for the person who has dementia. There are four modes of engagement relevant to enriched care planning which are presented in Table 6.1. Using this model to profile capacity for doing helps the person and their carer to identify their most comfortable mode of doing. This can give a helpful prediction of the types of 'doing' that will be manageable for the person.

In this part of the profiling process, you and the person you are profiling can use the Capacity for Doing Template to ascertain which doing skills are still intact and which are not and, from here, to identify the easiest mode of doing for the person.

The modes are described in Table 6.1 starting with the most basic and least demanding mode which is Automatic. The most demanding mode shown here is Goal Directed. In Allen's model, there are two further and more demanding modes which cognitively unimpaired adults can operate in described as 'Exploratory' and 'Planned'. These are not included here; in these modes, the person engages in abstract thinking; expresses complicated ideas; plans ahead; engages in demanding theoretical discussions, and weighs up probabilities and such like. Most of us operate in this mode for only short periods of time in a day. If we are tired, upset or ill, we will struggle to operate in this mode of doing.

Table 6.1 Modes of engagement

	Mode of engagement	Types of doing within this mode will include:
Skill 1: Turn head to look at object	*Automatic*	Gazing at objects, listening, feeling
Skill 2: Grasp object	*Postural*	Moving around, holding onto rails or furniture, pushing furniture; simple repetitive physical games (batting balloons) and exercise
Skill 3: Use hands to manipulate objects	*Manual*	Picking up, manipulating and moving objects
Skill 4: Begin to use simple tools		Rummaging, sorting and stacking objects; single-step tasks such as wiping, stirring, sweeping
Skill 5: Note effects of actions	*Goal-directed*	Matching objects, familiar multi-step daily living tasks
Skill 6: Sequence actions through known steps		

It is highly unlikely that a person who is ill or living with a chronic physical, mental or cognitive condition such as dementia will have a strong drive to be in these modes of doing.

This model is used by occupational therapists working in the field of dementia care (Perrin, May and Anderson 2008; Pool 2007) and has been developed more recently to make it useable for other carers (Pool 2007).

With this good practice guide, we offer a simple method for simple profiling of eating skills which can be used as an indicator of the person's capacity for doing. Preliminary trialling of this as a useable and reliable way for carers and professionals to understand enough about occupational capacity to better manage the person's care has been positive, but more work needs to be done for the future.

A person identified as being comfortable in the goal-directed mode of doing would most probably be able to eat independently using appropriate eating implements and using more than one eating implement at the same. However a person operating in the manual mode may struggle to use two implements and/or to use a knife for cutting; they may eat from their knife, cut with a spoon or a fork and/or eat with their fingers. In postural mode, the person would need more help, such as being given finger foods or help to hold a spoon or a cup and/or help to move the spoon or cup to their mouth. In the automatic mode, the person would need to be fed by another person.

Table 6.2 lists the actions you will be profiling using the Capacity for Doing Template and shows how these fit with Allen's model. The actions listed in the middle column are those listed on the Capacity for Doing Template. These are actions that the person tells you they can manage and/or that you observe.

USING THE CAPACITY FOR DOING PROFILING TEMPLATE

The Capacity for Doing Template is designed to help the person who has dementia and their carer(s) to understand what the person needs to remain fully engaged with the world. Abilities can be recognised and encouraged and help can be targeted in the right way. It offers a simple way of establishing or predicting the 'mode' in which the person with dementia engages with their world and has been adapted from the Cognitive Disabilities Model (Allen *et al.* 1992).

The template is completed in relation to the actions that the person is able to manage during eating and drinking. These can either be self-reported directly by the person or observed by the carer(s). Using the completed template makes it possible to establish an initial idea of the 'mode' that the person being profiled most comfortably adopts.

Table 6.2 Capacity for doing

The person does:	Predicted eating ability, as described on Capacity for Doing Template:	Allen's mode of engagement
Move body parts, engage through the senses Grasp object Use one object Differentiate between and use different objects Sustain action on objects Use objects with a goal in mind	Swallow Open mouth Turn head Drink from a cup placed in hand Pick up food with fingers Use one implement to eat Reach out and grasp one eating implement Cut food with one eating implement Separate, mash food with one eating implement Use two implements together to eat Use two implements together and cut food with knife	Goal-directed
Move body parts, engage through the senses Grasp object Use one object Differentiate between and use different objects Sustain action on objects	Swallow Open mouth Turn head Drink from a cup placed in hand Pick up food with fingers Use one implement to eat Reach out and grasp one eating implement Cut food with one eating implement Separate, mash food with one eating implement Use two implements together to eat	Manual
Move body parts, engage through the senses Grasp object Use one object Differentiate between and use different objects	Swallow Open Mouth Turn head Drink from a cup placed in hand Pick up food with fingers Use one implement to eat Reach out and grasp one eating implement	Manual
Move body parts, engage through the senses Grasp object	Swallow Open mouth Turn head Drink from a cup placed in hand	Postural

If the person being profiled has complex physical or mental health issues which interfere with his or her eating ability, this profiling tool may not be adequate, in which case a specialised assessment by an appropriately qualified and experienced occupational therapist is recommended.

Whether using observation or interview, it will be important to ensure that the person's true capacity is profiled. For example, it would be important to know that a person who is routinely fed by staff can pick up food and eat it without help. The feeding by staff in this instance is masking the capacity of the person with dementia. It may be necessary to set up independent situations for observing the person's abilities. For example, it might be appropriate during the observation to offer finger food outside of the normal mealtime routine to establish whether the person can pick up food or not.

By ticking each action that can be performed in sequence, starting with 'Turn my head' it should be possible to establish which mode of engagement the person predominantly uses. The 'I manage this well' ticks should run in sequence and come to a natural halt indicating whether the person's capacity for doing is primarily automatic, postural, manual or goal-directed.

Once you have an idea of which mode is comfortable for the person, you can use this in conjunction with the Capacity for Doing Support Guide shown below as Table 6.3 to develop a more Enriched Care Plan which details what the person needs in order to engage with their world and to exist as a 'doing' being.

IDENTIFYING AND DOCUMENTING NEEDS FROM THE CAPACITY FOR DOING PROFILE

Identifying needs

Identifying needs in relation to capacity for doing involves understanding which 'doing' skills are difficult or not possible for the person and which are easy and comfortable for the person to manage. The carer's role will be to support or compensate for the former and provide opportunities for the latter. Once you have identified the person's most comfortable mode of doing, you can use the guide below in Table 6.3 to identify needs. This is a shortened and simplified version of a more complex model which is described fully in *Wellbeing in Dementia: An Occupational Approach for Therapists and Carers* (Perrin and May 2008).

Table 6.3 Capacity for doing support guide

Most comfortable mode of doing:	Help will be needed to:	The environment should provide opportunities for engaging with:
Goal-directed	Plan ahead Manage new learning, new or unfamiliar environments and routines	Ordinary daily living activities, eating, self-care, games, sports, crafts, quizzes, end product tasks, talking and communicating, discussion, music, dance, drama, festivities, art, pottery and other creative activities, reminiscence, gardening, animals
Manual	Complete tasks such as daily living activities, eating, self-care	Talking and communicating, discussion, music, dance, drama, festivities, art, pottery and other creative activities, reminiscence, gardening, animals, sensory stimulation, rummaging, sorting, stacking, massage, exercise
Postural	Start off and keep going with daily living activities, eating and self-care; may need drink or spoon or other object to be placed in hand for the activity	Animals, sensory stimulation, rummaging, stacking, massage, exercise, balls/balloons, dolls, dressing up, moving around, pushing furniture
Automatic	Engage in a sensory way with the world through seeing, feeling, hearing, tasting	Animals, sensory stimulation, music, mobiles, smiling, rocking, singing or being sung to, non-verbal communication such as eye contact, smiling, soothing physical contact

Documenting needs

Having identified what is important for the person, you will now need to reflect this in what you write in the three working templates:

- Brief Profile Sheet
- Key Information Sheet
- The Enriched Care Plan.

Brief Profile Sheet

There is a space in the fifth section of the Brief Profile Sheet for circling the most comfortable mode of engagement for the person being profiled.

Key Information Sheet

Use the 'People that I may wish to contact' section to fill in names of anybody who is involved in helping the person to engage with their world such as their own occupational therapist, activity worker or volunteer.

The other section of relevance in the Key Information Sheet is further down the page and entitled 'Important information that I want people involved in my care to know about'. Again, if anything has come up during profiling of capacity for doing that the person feels is very important for others to know about, it can be recorded here. This might be something quite small but highly relevant, for example needing to use a teaspoon to eat, needing cup to be placed in hand in order to drink.

The Enriched Care Plan

The end product, the Enriched Care Plan, will be drawn from all the profiling that you do in relation to life story, lifestyle and future wishes, personality, health, capacity for doing, cognitive ability and life at the moment. There are just three columns in the plan. On the left hand side is the column entitled 'I need'. The middle column is headed 'My carers will'. The right hand column is for recording a date for review.

At this stage in the enriched care planning process, you only need write in the 'I need' column in relation to needs arising from capacity for doing. As already said, these needs will be things that make or break the person's day: things that are important *to* the person. Refer back to the Capacity for Doing Support Guide and use this just as a starting point. You will need to look at the suggested activities with the person and take into account their life story, lifestyle, personality and health before coming up with a tailored 'list' of needs.

Here are some examples of what you might write in the Enriched Care Plan:

> *I need:*
>
> - gentle verbal encouragement to finish daily tasks such as eating and dressing
>
> - items to be handed to me one at a time
>
> - opportunities to exercise by walking every day
>
> - opportunities to take part in sports discussions and quizzes
>
> - opportunities to see, touch and smell fresh flowers.

SUMMARY

- For the person with dementia 'doing' can become difficult or even impossible but it is never the case that any person (unless in a coma) is completely unable to engage with their world.

- Engagement is a broad term for all the things we do to connect with the world around us ranging from gazing at objects or people right through to the more complex types of doing such as driving a car or cooking a meal.

- People who have dementia seem to be particularly at risk of not 'doing' or of becoming disengaged and this can lead to ill-being.

- The capacity for doing profiling process helps you and the person being profiled to find out about their most comfortable mode of doing.

- The Enriched Care Plan provides clear actions that the carer needs to take to help the person to engage with their world.

Chapter 7

Cognitive Ability

Taking cognitive support needs on board as a whole workforce issue is an important development in dementia care. This is the one area that has been under-developed in provision of education and training for people who have dementia and their carers. While it is true that knowledge and expertise in relation to dementia and the brain and behaviour continues to increase among medical professionals, there is still a great deal of ignorance and misinformation about this at ground level where arguably, it is most needed.

Common misconceptions are that dementia is:

- just part of getting old

- going mad in old age

- when you imagine things and get paranoid

- having a bad memory

- a hopeless disease for which there is no cure

- tragic because nothing can be done.

This kind of thinking results in care that is inadequate when in fact there is much that can be done to provide cognitive support as well as physical, social and psychological support. Ignoring cognitive support needs means closing the door to numerous practical interventions that can do much to promote well-being.

Profiling cognitive ability is not intended to replace standardised cognitive assessments which have a place and a value in dementia care; however, we firmly believe that there is a straightforward body of knowledge about cognitive issues in dementia that can be easily transferred into the knowledge set of the dementia care workforce at large. This section provides information to underpin that knowledge. The Cognitive Ability Template brings to light any cognitive impairment that the person has or may have. In the final section of this chapter, we will look at how to indentify and document needs arising from this profile. Meeting these cognitive needs will become an important part of the enriched plan.

DEMENTIA AND THE BRAIN

Two of the most common causes of dementia, especially in older people, are Alzheimer's disease and vascular dementia (Alzheimer's Society 2008). Both of these conditions cause damage to the cortex of the brain. The cortex is the outer surface of the brain. It is about one eighth of an inch in thickness and contains billions of neurons and synaptic connections. The folds in the cortex increase the surface area allowing room for more neurons and more activity between them. This outer layer of brain makes it possible for us to learn to do all the things that we can't do as a newborn baby. These are called acquired skills.

Different parts of the cortex are responsible for the different 'jobs' the human brain needs to do in order to perform these acquired skills. They are 'cognitive' jobs i.e. to do with brainwork and each job takes part in a specific area of the cortex.

Broadly speaking, the jobs can be divided up into four main types:

- visual processing

- body management and integration of physical experiences

- memory and auditory processing

- planning, judging and controlling.

Alzheimer's disease and vascular dementia are just two of a number of conditions that damage the cortex of the brain making it difficult or impossible for some of these jobs to be done.

Each lobe has a job to do:

> Occipital lobe: visual processing

> Parietal lobe: body management and integration of physical experiences

> Temporal lobe: auditory processing, language and words, memory

> Frontal lobe: higher intellectual functioning, planning, judging, controlling

Figure 7.1 shows the left view of the cortex. This is a very simplified explanation of the brain and behaviour. For more detail see Chapter 1 of Perrin and May 2008.

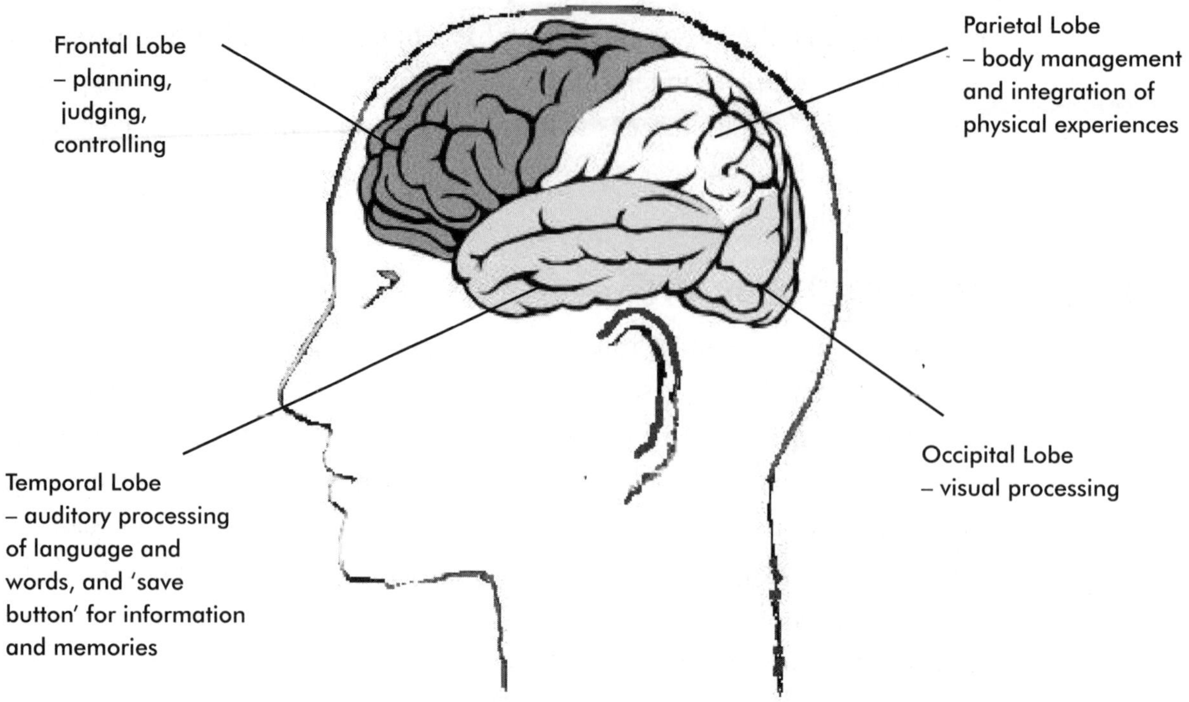

Frontal Lobe
– planning,
judging,
controlling

Parietal Lobe
– body management
and integration of
physical experiences

Occipital Lobe
– visual processing

Temporal Lobe
– auditory processing
of language and
words, and 'save
button' for information
and memories

Figure 7.1: A view of the cortex from the left

Visual processing

Visual processing enables us to make sense of the images that the eyes bring to our cortex and it takes place in the occipital lobe. If there is damage here, the person will need help to make sense of visual images.

Visual difficulties caused by damage to the occipital lobe include:

- visual blind spots which may cause a person to bump into furniture

- problems seeing lines, edges, shapes

- problems seeing colour

- problems seeing movement

- problems seeing depth.

Body management and integration of physical experiences

When our parietal lobe is doing its job, the body moves around efficiently and effortlessly. This part of the cortex enables us to know, for example, where our feet are and how they feel without having to look at them or physically touch them; to lean back in our chair until our back finds the back of the chair without feeling as though we are falling; to know where we are in a room and where the room is in a house. If there is damage in this region, problems in performing everyday activities may be experienced including:

- difficulties with skilled actions (e.g. using cutlery, getting dressed)

- problems scanning the environment

- poor awareness of body position

- problems with reading, writing, numbers.

Auditory processing of language and words and our 'save button' for information and memories

Alzheimer's disease typically damages the temporal lobe and this part of the cortex is where we process what we hear and save and file new information and memories. When the temporal lobe is damaged certain difficulties result including:

- declining general knowledge, especially of fine detail and less familiar subjects

- language difficulties

- difficulties with word-finding

- problems understanding what others say

- problems recognising objects

- problems recognising people

- problems recognising places

- memory loss.

There is a very important structure underneath this part of the cortex called the hippocampus. The hippocampus makes it possible for us to update what we store in our memory with new information. The hippocampus is affected very early on in the progression of Alzheimer's disease and it is rather like our brain's 'save button'. If it isn't working properly, memories about daily events are lost as quickly as they occur. This results in the person failing to update their knowledge about how the world around them is changing. For example how their familiar friends and family are changing physically over time; how a microwave works; what a modern telephone looks like. The person has to draw on what they have 'saved' i.e. old memories and knowledge to make sense of what is happening around them. This is why some people mistake their son for their husband or don't recognise their own reflection in the mirror or believe themselves to be in a certain place.

Planning, judging, controlling

These are the 'higher' acquired skills which are the last to develop. It is the proper functioning of this area at the front part of the cortex, the frontal lobe, that enables us to plan what we want to do; weigh up and understand the consequences of what we do; think in the abstract; and control our primitive thoughts and feelings so that our behaviour is acceptable in the social world. There is a particular type of dementia that affects this specific part of the cortex called 'fronto-temporal dementia'.

Some people who have vascular dementia may also have damage in this area. Problems associated with frontal lobe damage include:

- repetitive actions

- poor concentration

- poor planning/inefficient behaviour

- inability to prioritise

- inability to sequence events

- loss of any care/concerns for others

- rash and impulsive behaviour

- rudeness

- rule breaking

- sexual disinhibition

- aggression.

The brain as an entire system

This has been a very simplified and short explanation of how the cortex works and the implications for the person when certain cognitive 'jobs' cannot be done. One last important aspect to mention is that these different parts of the brain do not operate in isolation – they connect with each other and work together, as a system. So, if one job isn't being done in the same way, the rest of the system is affected and this can cause:

- confusion

- hallucinations

- delusions

- mis-identifications

- false beliefs

- reality drifting into the past.

Alzheimer's disease causes plaques and tangles to form, initially in the temporal area, but eventually these find their way into the rest of the brain. So initial cognitive support needs for a person who has Alzheimer's disease will be to do with language and memory. As time goes by, the person will need more support with additional cognitive problems relating to body management, visual processing, planning, judging and controlling.

Vascular dementia causes cell death by loss of oxygen to parts of the brain. This can happen when blood vessels to and within the brain are blocked, or they burst. Vascular dementia does not follow a set pattern; the cell death can happen in several different places over a period of time. This makes it inappropriate to use a 'stage theory' for dementia because of the individualised and *ad hoc* nature of cerebral vascular disease.

The three most important messages about cognitive support needs for a person who has dementia are:

- They can change over time.

- They are highly individual.

- They are guaranteed to involve more than memory alone.

USING THE COGNITIVE ABILITY PROFILING TEMPLATE

This template guides the person who has dementia and/or their carer(s) through a detailed consideration of all of the cognitive 'jobs' that need to be done and how well the person is managing them. This enables the provision of tailored support, which it is hoped will reduce the extent of the person's disability. For example, knowing that a person struggles to recognise objects would result in a care plan that includes directions to staff to name objects when presenting them to the person.

Using this template is likely to take some time; the person being profiled will need support to consider the cognitive difficulties they are experiencing and the carer(s) may need to make observations of the person in order to understand these experiences. The most useful observations will be of the person engaging in day-to-day activities such as eating, dressing and communicating with others.

The template has five sections:

- Visual Processing

- Body Management and Awareness

- Memory

- Communication

- Planning, Judging and Controlling.

Within each section there are several specific statements aimed at finding out if the person has any difficulties. For each question, there are four options, one of which you should tick.

The options are:

- This happens to me sometimes

- This doesn't happen to me

- I'm not sure

- Please ask my carer.

You should only tick one column for each statement. Ticks in the 'This happens to me sometimes' column flag up cognitive support needs which you should carry forward to the Enriched Care Plan. Ticks in the 'I'm not sure' or 'Please ask my carer' columns mean that further work needs to be done in order to find out if there is a cognitive support need. This too needs to be documented in the care plan. As always, it is good practice to seek consent from the person to look in their notes, make your own observations or consult other carers. It is also good practice to share your findings with the person, giving an explanation as to why this is significant for them and their care.

Visual Processing

I see only part of what is in front of me

If the person being profiled sees only part of what is in front of them, this will cause difficulties for them in most activities of daily living such as eating, washing, dressing, moving about as well as socialising. This difficulty can also pose safety risks, for example an increased risk of bumping into or tripping over things and a risk of poor nutrition through only eating parts of meals. However, it is unlikely that the person will be able to report this as a problem. Most people who have this problem don't know it – they simply see their world differently. If the person is seeing only part of what is in front of them, you can pick this up either by observing and spending time with the person or from information recorded in medical, cognitive or other assessment reports.

I see things that other people don't see

This refers to hallucinations. It is unlikely that a person experiencing visual hallucinations will report them as such because they are real to them. However, they may experience not being believed by others or report that it is others who can't see properly.

Sometimes dementia causes hallucinations and these become part of what the person believes to be real and no amount of persuasion will change what they believe. More importantly, the person may feel frightened or anxious or driven to act in some way in response to their hallucinations. The person's feelings should be acknowledged and supported and genuine offers of help made. It is possible to work with a person's feelings and at the same time to be honest about the fact that their reality is different from yours.

For example, James would sometimes become very worried that he was 'in trouble'. He would explain that he'd seen somebody in his room and that they were after him for something. His carer would say 'I can see you're worried, James, shall I go and check your room and see if anybody is there now?' His carer was then able to report back to him honestly that nobody was there now. She was also able to tell him that she would help him out again if there were any more problems.

I find it hard to find the object I am looking for, even when it is right in front of me

This is a common cognitive problem, especially in strange, poorly lit or visually overcrowded environments. It can stop a person from getting on with simple jobs such as eating a meal or getting dressed and washed in the morning. The person may well tell you that they have this difficulty but you might also observe it.

Everyday objects look strange or unrecognisable

This is more likely to be something you observe. You can find out if this is a problem by spending time with the person while they are handling objects such as hair brushes, pens, cups and noting whether or not they are using the object properly. It is not uncommon for a person who has difficulty with visual processing to become tense or frightened when faced with something that looks strange. For example, a blue shiny floor might look like water and cause a person to stop in their tracks and not wish to step on it.

Body Management and Awareness

It is difficult for me to start getting dressed or undressed on my own without someone to prompt me

> Getting dressed and undressed, like many daily living activities, are 'multi-step' tasks. This means that there are several steps involved in completing the task. It is not uncommon for a person to have difficulty just with starting off the sequence of steps. So, as part of the profiling process you may want to try prompting the person to begin the task. This can be done verbally – 'Would you like to start getting dressed now?' – or non-verbally e.g. showing the item of clothing to the person, or laying their clothes out in sequence on the bed. If, after the prompt, the person manages to get on and complete the rest of the task then the difficulty is pinpointed to one to do with starting off.

It is difficult for me to choose my clothes from my wardrobe/dresser spontaneously

> There may be a number of reasons for a person having difficulty choosing their clothes. It might just be that they can't find where their clothes are. Or choosing between more than two items is too difficult, in which case the person will need to be presented with just two items at a time to choose from. If, when presented with just two items, the person still struggles, they may need you to decide on their behalf using information from their life story and lifestyle. Or, perhaps there are other issues such as visual problems or difficulty understanding what is being asked which should come to light as you go through the enriched profiling process.

It is difficult for me to co-ordinate my arms and body parts during washing or dressing

> If the person cannot integrate all that is happening to and around them, they may not be able to move and co-ordinate themselves in the most efficient way for activities such as washing and dressing. If this seems to be a problem it will be important to reduce the demands upon the person by limiting the noise and activity around them; give 'single step' instructions such as 'lift your arm' and touch or pat the body part that you are asking the person to move.

It is difficult for me to know exactly where my arms or legs are during washing or dressing

If this is the case, you may need to move with and for the person. This means lifting their arms and legs with and for them during self-care activities. It is usually helpful to adopt a running commentary as you do this which is talking the person through what is happening. Again, keep noise and activity around the person to a minimum, work with one body part at a time and work at a pace that is comfortable for the person.

Memory

I have difficulty remembering what I have seen

If the person you are profiling often forgets family visits, TV programmes they have watched, or written notes then it is likely that they have a poor visual memory. This is important to know because using visual cues such as leaving notes won't necessarily be a useful support intervention in this case.

I have difficulty remembering what has been said to me

Forgetting conversations is a sign that the person has a poor auditory memory. Again this is important to know so as to avoid implementing unhelpful strategies and interventions in the Enriched Care Plan.

I have difficulty recognising faces of people I know

Familiar friends and family members usually report that their loved one no longer recognises them if this happens. Another sign that this may be an issue is if the person talks to their own image in the mirror as if it were another person.

I have difficulty recognising familiar objects

It is important not to assume that the person sees and recognises objects in the same way as you do. A pen, cup or watch for example may not look familiar for a person who has dementia. A simple way of supporting the person is to get into the habit of always naming all objects as you hand them to the person. For example, 'Here is your pen', 'Here is your cup', 'Here is your watch'. This may ease the strain of struggling to recognise familiar objects.

I have difficulty recognising familiar surroundings

Getting lost in *familiar* surroundings can be a sign of memory difficulties and will give rise to a cognitive support need. Making sure the person carries something to identify them is one of several ways of supporting a person who is at risk of getting lost in their own living environment or community.

I have difficulty remembering the layout of where I am

This is a different type of difficulty requiring a different kind of support. Being unable to learn a new layout is probably more common and specially adapted environments using signs, colour and such like can really reduce the stress and anxiety induced by feelings of being lost.

I have difficulty remembering where I have put things

Losing things is common but frustrating and disabling and needs to be flagged up if it is a problem. Providing support is important in keeping people active and calm.

Communication

Below are brief descriptions of some of the commonly experienced communication difficulties associated with having dementia. To develop a more in-depth understanding and find out about a wider range of things you can do to help, we recommend you read *Care to Communicate* (Powell 2000).

I have difficulty starting off talking

Just because a person isn't saying much doesn't mean they have nothing to say. Introducing a theme or asking a question are both good ways to help a person to start talking. The more you know about the person's life story the better position you will be in to use themes, topics, objects pictures etc. that are meaningful for the individual.

I have difficulty stopping talking

This is sometimes called perseveration which means repetition of a word, phrase, gesture or action. The person keeps on going regardless of what changes around them and may need help to stop. If the person you are profiling tends to talk for long uninterrupted periods in a repetitive way, this can be a cognitive issue. Although this is unlikely to be a problem for the person, the reactions of others around them can become negative in which case you may need to find ways of protecting the person from such responses.

It is difficult for me to reply when people talk to me

There may be a number of reasons why this is happening, including:

- The person talking is saying too much too quickly.

- The person talking is not allowing enough time for a response.

- The type of response being asked for is too difficult, for example the response to 'Would you like custard or ice cream now?' is easier to respond to than 'What would you like for your sweet after dinner tomorrow? Here's the menu.'

- The person talking wants a spoken response when a nod or shake of the head would be easier.

- The words can't be heard.

- The words can't be understood.

I lose track of what I am talking about

This happens to us all sometimes, usually when we have too many things on our mind, or when we are tired or when something distracts us. Often, having someone recap what we have said so far helps us to get back on track. This strategy can also be useful for a person whose cognitive impairment is causing them to lose track. The most important thing is to keep the communication going with nods and eye contact; you can steer the person back on track but if this disrupts the flow too much it can be better to keep going with the next theme.

I can't think of the word I want

Again, this happens to us all sometimes and being helped to find the word often solves the problem. Don't keep on with this though if the flow of the communication is being disrupted too much or you are making the person feel inept.

It is difficult for me to understand what is being said to me

This isn't always as easy to recognise as a problem. If the person being profiled struggles to follow the plot in TV dramas or seems to switch off in group discussions, these may be signs that they are having difficulty converting the sounds of words into meaningful language. If this is recognised by the person themselves or by you the carer as a problem, you will need to adapt the way you communicate to make it easier. Strategies for this include:

- Using concrete language and avoiding the use of concepts e.g. 'Would you like to see some flowers?' is a concrete question and easier to process than 'Would you like to come to the garden centre?'

- Using chunks of information i.e. give a brief summary or gist rather than a long drawn-out story e.g. 'Your daughter has phoned to say she'll be here in an hour' is easier to process than 'Your daughter phoned to apologise for not getting here sooner but her car has broken down and she is waiting for a friend to come and get her and then she's got to pick up the children so she can't get here until tea time.'

- Using gestures instead of words or alongside words e.g. waving to say hello or goodbye, thumbs up to signal yes, thumbs down to signal no.

Planning, Judging and Controlling

I find it difficult to focus on what I want to do

This is sometimes referred to as 'attention', the ability to block out anything irrelevant so as to focus on the task at hand. This might be background noise or activity, or thoughts and feelings that are distracting. A person who is less able to do this will really struggle to stay focused on what they set out to do. They may, for example, set off to get something and then get distracted *en route* and start off a different task altogether and so on through the day. This needn't be a problem for the person as long as the end result does not cause them harm. If they are neglecting vital jobs or becoming disengaged socially as a result, they may need carer support to compensate for this cognitive impairment.

It is difficult for me to plan ahead

Forward planning is often an activity that people need help with. This might be in relation to big things like holidays, organising gifts and cards for birthdays and Christmas; or it can be for much smaller but no less important day-to-day things like what to wear, what to eat, when to start getting ready for bed.

Supporting Parietal Lobe Function

- Touch and name body parts when assisting
- Gently pat small of back before and during physical assistance
- Help to direct gaze in the right place
- Help to complete dressing, washing
- Help to maintain comfortable and safe body posture
- Slow down when assisting

Supporting Frontal Lobe Function:

- Talk about what needs to be done today/tomorrow (planning)
- Talk about anticipated problems
- Talk about the likely consequences for chosen actions (judging)
- Give clear verbal and non-verbal signals, messages and responses (controlling)

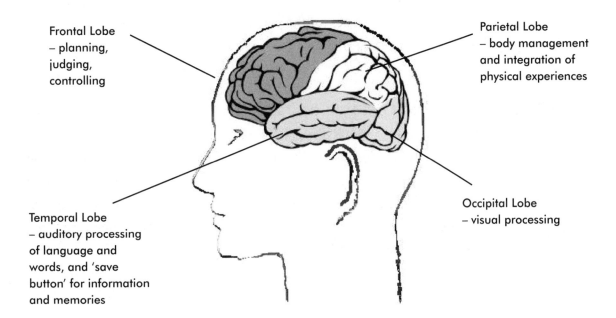

Frontal Lobe – planning, judging, controlling

Parietal Lobe – body management and integration of physical experiences

Temporal Lobe – auditory processing of language and words, and 'save button' for information and memories

Occipital Lobe – visual processing

Supporting Occipital Lobe Function

- Use colours to help to distinguish object; dark on light background or light on dark background
- Name objects when presenting them
- Present objects at eye level – within 15–20 cm
- Avoid shiny flooring
- Avoid heavily patterned flooring
- Use classic shaped objects and furniture
- Use uplift lighting to avoid shadows
- Make objects needed visible
- Be aware of areas of visual inattention or blind spots
- Remove objects not needed from eyeshot
- Pay extra attention to lighting

Supporting Temporal Lobe Function

- Repeat information as often as needed in a positive relaxed manner
- Adopt a running commentary when assisting
- Use simple concrete language
- Know as much as possible about what is stored in the person's memory
- Give 'safe' verbal and non-verbal signals
- Provide environmental cues telling of the place, time of day, time of year

Figure 7.2 Universal procedures for supporting cognitive function

I find it difficult to learn anything new

How many redundant microwaves, new televisions, music systems and such like are lying around in people's houses having never been used? Family members often buy these things to help and make life easier for their older relative. The fact is though, that using new gadgets requires a person to learn how to operate them. This is new learning and can be difficult for a person who has dementia.

If new learning is difficult or not possible, carers need to try to make sure that the person can go about their day-to-day lives safely, comfortably and enjoyably without the need to learn anything new. So carers need to know if this is a problem but also be able to act for the person recognising situations that require new learning and helping the person to avoid or get through these.

It is difficult for me to start off on a course of action

As with talking, this can be a distinct cognitive impairment – often leading to the person being judged to be unwilling or unable to do anything. A person who has difficulty starting off actions and activities needs somebody or something else to do this for them. Carers can help by using verbal encouragement or providing non-verbal prompts such as touch, gesture or even giving associated objects to the person such as a brush to start off brushing hair or a flannel to start off washing.

It is difficult for me to stop what I am doing

The term 'perseveration' was mentioned earlier in relation to stopping talking. Well, the same thing can happen in relation to doing and it can cause a person to keep doing the same thing over and over repetitively. Walking, picking things up, rocking backwards and forwards are some of the actions that people might do repetitively. Again, you should only need to regard this as a problem if it is causing harm or ill-being for the person themselves. Examples of this might be if the person is becoming dehydrated or exhausted as a result of keeping going with an action or an activity, or causing other people to get angry and strike out. If harm is being caused, you will need to treat it as a need and move it forward into the Enriched Care Plan.

I have trouble controlling my emotions

This can be a problem for a person who has frontal lobe damage. This can cause the person to seem to change perhaps from being a polite reserved character to being somebody who shouts or swears a lot. It is perfectly human and normal for all of us to experience a range of emotions some of which might be quite strong. However, our frontal lobes enable us to manage these feelings; we can make a judgement about whether to show our feelings or not; we can know what the implications of our actions or words will be and we can remember previous times when we've had the feelings and how we have managed them. All of these cognitive abilities make it possible for us to control our emotions. A person for whom these abilities no longer come easy may behave more impulsively and may show strong emotions more freely.

I have trouble controlling my impulses

Similarly, frontal lobe damage returns us to primitive 'in the moment' behaviour which is to act without thinking in an impulsive fashion. Examples we have seen include taking clothes off when hot, eating handfuls of food, sometimes belonging to other people when hungry, hitting out when frightened or confused.

IDENTIFIYING AND DOCUMENTING NEEDS FROM THE COGNITIVE ABILITY PROFILE

Identifying needs

Much of the work involved in identifying cognitive support needs will have already been done during the profiling process. If you have ticked in the columns 'This happens to me sometimes', 'I'm not sure' or, 'Please ask my carer' anywhere on the profile, this needs to be carried forward and documented as a need in the Enriched Care Plan. Cognitive jobs which the person isn't sure about or for which they have requested that you ask their carer need to be considered further and this too needs to be recorded in the Enriched Care Plan.

When you have finished profiling the person's cognitive ability and support needs, you can use Figure 7.2 to help you to identify supportive carer interventions. However, because cognitive impairment is so difficult to pinpoint fully and precisely for each individual, we strongly recommend a workforce approach to supporting people. This requires every worker in a care setting to adopt the interventions in Figure 7.2 as 'universal procedures' when working with populations of people who have cognitive support needs. Universal procedures are standardised, routine ways of working; they are used all the time, with every person. The idea is that these ways of working will provide support to those who need it and cause no harm or offence to those who don't.

An overarching principle for supporting a person who is experiencing the world differently is that of believing. The principle of believing is that the carer believes that what the person is experiencing is real to them. This enables the carer to acknowledge and validate the person's feelings even when reality for each is different. This becomes very important when, for example, the person is experiencing hallucinations. Identifying and working with feelings is part of providing cognitive support.

Documenting needs

Having established the needs of the person in relation to their cognitive profile you will now need to reflect these in what you write in the three working templates:

- Brief Profile Sheet
- Key Information Sheet
- The Enriched Care Plan.

Brief Profile Sheet

There is a space in the sixth section of the Brief Profile Sheet for circling cognitive support needs that have come to light through profiling.

Key Information Sheet

Use the 'People that I may wish to contact' section to fill in names of anybody who has been or is involved in the cognitive aspects of the person's care such as the name of their key worker, neurologist, geriatrician psychologist, occupational therapist, speech therapist or any other specialist.

The other section of relevance in the Key Information Sheet is further down the page and entitled 'Important information that I want people involved in my care to know about'. Again, if anything has come up during profiling of cognitive ability that the person feels is very important for others to know about, it can be recorded here. This might be in relation to needing information to be repeated or to be offered choices in a certain way.

The Enriched Care Plan

The end product, the Enriched Care Plan, will be drawn from all the profiling that you do in relation to life story, lifestyle and future wishes, personality, health, capacity for doing, cognitive ability and life at the moment. There are just three columns in the plan. On the left hand side is the column entitled 'I need'. The middle column is headed 'My carers will'. The right hand column is for recording a date for review.

At this stage in the enriched care planning process, you only need write in the 'I need' column in relation to needs arising from cognitive support issues. Drawing from the actual Cognitive Ability Template, here are some examples of what you might record in this column:

I need

- help to process what I see

  - people and objects to be placed in my left field of vision
  - objects to be named when you give them to me
  - to be believed when I see things that you don't see

- help with body management and integration of physical experience

  - to be patted in the small of my back when I am moving from one place to another

- help to compensate for my poor memory

  - people, even those familiar to me, to tell me their name and their relationship to me each time they speak to me

- understanding that I find it difficult to control my impulses

  - people around me to give clear messages to me about what I can and cannot do.

SUMMARY

- Cognitive support is one area that has been poorly understood in caring for people who have dementia.

- Dementia most commonly affects the cortex of the brain which is responsible for all the skills we learn to do after birth.

- These include visual processing, body management and integration of physical experiences, auditory processing, language and memory, higher intellectual functioning, reasoning, planning, judging and controlling.

- It is with these skills that the person who has dementia may need support.

- The three most important messages about cognitive support needs for a person who has dementia are:

  ○ they change over time
  ○ they are highly individual
  ○ they are guaranteed to involve more than memory alone.

- The capacity for doing profiling process involves finding out which skills the person needs help with.

- The Enriched Care Plan includes practical steps that the carer can take to reduce disability caused by cognitive impairment.

Chapter 8

Life at the Moment

This last but crucially important part of the profiling process is about exploring issues relating to the person's experience of life at the moment which may be having an affect on their well-being. We know, from what people with dementia say and from what we have observed, that the quality of life at the moment is profoundly affected by other people and the 'feel' of the social environment in which we live.

> How you relate to us has a big impact on the course of the disease. You can restore our personhood, and give us a sense of being needed and valued. There is a Zulu saying that is very true. 'A person is a person through others'. Give us reassurance, hugs, support, a meaning in life. (Bryden 2005, p.127)

For any person, living permanently in a world where feelings of isolation, dissatisfaction, confusion, frustration and fear are ignored would be intolerable.

There is still an out-of-date prejudice that people who have dementia can't express their opinion. But this is not true:

> It's as though that's it, you are dribbling and nodding, and that's Alzheimer's. That's the picture of Alzheimer's. But we are all sitting here talking perfectly normally. We have got Alzheimer's of some form, we are not nodding and dribbling. (person with dementia) (Alzheimer's Society 2008, p.45)

The first section of the Life at the Moment Template provides spaces for writing down what the person and significant others say they feel about their life at the moment. The person being profiled is encouraged to talk about how they feel about their life at the moment. Views from an advocate who might be a family member or friend can also be recorded to supplement what the person is communicating about how he or she is feeling.

Planning and giving care without any recognition of the person's 'experience' can lead to a style of caring that objectifies the person. This template is designed to help the carer to seek out and listen to the person receiving their care and to develop an approach to care planning that is inclusive and collaborative.

Underpinning the whole Enriched Model is a belief that the 'social psychology' component of the equation is very powerful in its effect on the experience of dementia. This means that the extent to which the person experiences well- or ill-being is largely down to how it feels for them to be where they are – more so even than how 'severe' their dementia is. Living a life feeling bad inside causes ill-being and ill-being can spiral downwards pulling physical health and ability to function in the world down with it.

We all have unpleasant episodes in our lives which cause us to feel bad inside but, in the absence of cognitive impairment, we are able to process negative feelings. We can do this by acting in the situation to change it, leaving the situation, talking and thinking about it afterwards, using logic to come to terms with what has happened, understand what has happened and move on. Having dementia can interfere with or prevent this important 'processing' and the risk then is that the feelings stay with the person and cause harm.

We all know that how life feels for us in the moment is largely down to the quality of our relationships with other people; the extent to which we are socially involved and accepted and how engaged or disengaged we are generally with the world around us.

In working with carers to improve person-centred care we use Kitwood's flower shown below in Figure 8.1 (Kitwood 1997) to help us to look at this.

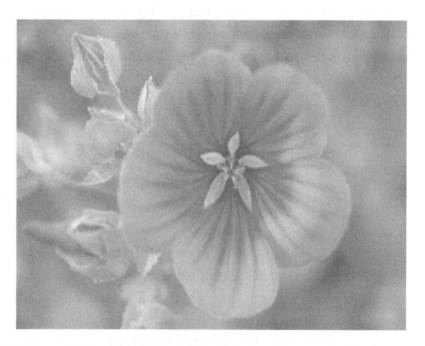

Figure 8.1: Kitwood's flower representing psychological needs

The flower has five petals each of which represents a psychological need. The needs are:

- comfort

- occupation

- attachment

- identity

- inclusion.

The second section of the Life at the Moment Template, 'My Psychological Needs', has been designed to help you and the person you are profiling to explore the extent to which the needs are being met. This model is used by people who have been trained to use Dementia Care Mapping to profile the overall nature of how their care is experienced by the recipient(s) which helps to develop carers' awareness of the impact on the person of a strong, psychologically supportive environment.

There is a third tool that we recommend for use alongside the enriched care planning Life at the Moment Template and this is the Bradford Well Being Profile which is published by and available from the Bradford Dementia Group (Bradford Dementia Group 2008). It has been developed over several years and is designed to help carers to monitor the well-being of individual clients in their care on an ongoing basis. You can use it to contribute to the enriched care planning process and it can also be used as a way of keeping track of how well or not the Enriched Care Plan is working, of how a person is fairing over time.

USING THE LIFE AT THE MOMENT PROFILING TEMPLATE
These are my feelings, about living my life here

It may or may not be the best thing to set up a special interview to find out how the person feels about their life. You will need to decide what suits the person best; it may be that a combination of 'interview' style, time and informal chats will work. Remember though that, very often, the most true and meaningful expressions of satisfaction or dissatisfaction come during informal discussions. You should write down here, with permission, anything significant that the person says, or things that they do to show approval or disapproval about what is happening around them and to them, particularly anything that can be addressed and improved upon by the carer(s). There is a real art to communicating in a safe and non-judgemental way and we recommend that, if you are interested in and motivated to improve your communication skills, you read *Communication and Consultation: Exploring Ways for Staff to Involve People with Dementia in Developing Services* (Allan 2001).

When talking about general satisfaction, it is best to ask, in the moment if possible, about feelings rather than facts. For example, if you want to know how satisfied a person is with the food you should ask during or just after the meal. Ask how the food tastes rather than what the food is or was. Do you like the flavour, the texture, is it hot enough? The same principle applies to exploring levels of satisfaction about the building, the people and the care that is given. The words you use will need to be tailored to suit the individual, but here is a list of the topics you may wish to explore together:

- staying here forever

- feeling hot or cold or just right, during the day and at night

- feeling comfy in the bed, or chair

- feeling safe when alone, and with other people

- liking the staff, not liking the staff

- liking the other residents, not liking them

- liking or not liking the amount of fresh air and light

- liking or not liking the furniture or carpets

- liking or not liking how people talk to me

- liking or not liking the taste of the food

- feeling hungry or thirsty in the day and at night

- liking or not liking the clothes I wear.

If the person you are profiling struggles to understand you or to be understood by you, it may be appropriate to work with a family member or advocate and there is a space in the right hand box for recording what others say on behalf of the person.

My psychological needs

The purpose of this part of the template is to identify those needs that are not being adequately met for the person so that unmet or poorly met needs can be carried forward into their Enriched Care Plan. Talking about psychological needs must be approached gently and with sensitivity in a manner that is comfortable and manageable for the person. You may need to use your own judgement as well your observations and use information given by other people you have talked to in order to gain an overall 'feel' for how the person is faring psychologically. In our experience, using the actual words 'comfort', 'occupation', 'attachment', 'identity', 'inclusion' in direct conversation with the person is not helpful. There are other more understandable words that you can use, as in the following questions.

Comfort

- Do you feel loved and looked after here?
- Do you feel safe inside or a bit wobbly?
- Are you warm enough?
- Do you have any pain?
- Do you feel you can relax?
- What happens when you feel upset?
- Is there somewhere you can go or somebody to talk to when you feel worried or upset?

Occupation

- Do you ever get bored?
- Are you busy enough here?
- Is there anything you would like to be doing?
- Are you ever stopped from doing what you want?
- Are there any special things you need to keep close to you so that you can hold or look at them whenever you want – like pictures, books?
- Is there anything I can do to help you feel useful and active?

Attachment

- Do you think about your mother and father ever?
- Are there other people that you miss?
- What do you do to feel close to them?
- Is there a special person that you carry around with you in your memory?
- Do you have a special friend here?
- Do you have a special belonging that you keep with you, for security?

Identity

- Do you think they know the real you here?
- Are these your clothes, do you like them?
- Have you got your own special belongings here with you?
- Do people here understand your sense of humour?
- Do they know about your family and your life story?

Inclusion

- Do other people like you here?
- Do they do things, activities and such like, here?
- Do they ask you to join in?
- Do you want to join in?
- Do you ever feel left out?
- Do you feel part of the group?

IDENTIFYING AND DOCUMENTING NEEDS FROM THE LIFE AT THE MOMENT PROFILE

Identifying needs

Needs in relation to life at the moment will relate to those areas of life that are causing dissatisfaction and psychological needs that are not being met adequately. Any dissatisfaction expressed during the profiling process needs to be looked at carefully with a view to putting it right. For example, if not liking the food is an area of dissatisfaction, enjoying food will need to be moved forward as a need in the Enriched Care Plan. Any psychological need that has a tick in the 'Minimally and/or infrequently met' or the 'Not met at all' boxes will need also to be carried forward as a need. If there are no ticks in these columns, then you should look at the 'Moderately or sometimes met' column and move these needs forward into the Enriched Care Plan.

Documenting needs

Having identified the needs the person has to improve their experience of life at the moment, you will now need to reflect this in what you write in the three working templates:

- Brief Profile Sheet

- Key Information Sheet

- The Enriched Care Plan.

Brief Profile Sheet

There is a space in the seventh section of the Brief Profile Sheet to record significant issues for immediate attention. These should be serious or major needs that are more likely to be met if known about by the wider care team. For example if the person has said they often feel left out, or if they are suffering because they are missing somebody so much.

Key Information Sheet

Use the 'People that I may wish to contact' section to fill in names of anybody who makes a real difference to the person's quality of life at the moment. This could be a family member, a friend and/or a member of the care team. The other section of relevance in the Key Information Sheet is further down the page and entitled 'Important information that I want people involved in my care to know about'. Again, if anything has come up during profiling of life at the moment that the person feels is very important for others to know about, it can be recorded here. This might be in relation to something within the care setting that is causing major discomfort or a recent bereavement or loss.

The Enriched Care Plan

The end product, the Enriched Care Plan, will be drawn from all the profiling that you do in relation to life story, lifestyle and future wishes, personality, health, capacity for doing, cognitive ability and life at the moment. There are just three columns in the plan. On the left hand side is the column entitled 'I need'. The middle column is headed 'My carers will'. The right hand column is for recording a date for review.

At this stage in the enriched care planning process, you only need write in the 'I need' column in relation to needs arising from cognitive ability and cognitive support issues.

Drawing from the actual Life at the Moment Template, here are some examples of what you might record in this column:

I need

- to feel warm at night
- to be included in social activities
- to keep my handbag with me all the time
- to talk about my wife sometimes
- for other people to know about my childhood
- help to find my knitting and do some every day.

SUMMARY

- Our quality of life at the moment is profoundly affected by how other people treat us and the 'feel' of the social environment in which we live.

- One way of profiling quality of life is to look at our psychological needs for comfort, occupation, attachment, identity and inclusion.

- The life at the moment profiling process provides a structure for looking at how satisfied generally the person is with their life at the moment and the extent to which these psychological needs are being met.

- The Enriched Care Plan addresses poorly met psychological needs with clear action to be taken by the carer to improve matters.

Chapter 9

Implementing and Reviewing the Enriched Care Plan

This is the final and the shortest chapter in this good practice guide about enriched care planning. How well you implement and review care plans will depend very much on the value and importance given to this process in your work setting. Very often, staff tell us that they have little involvement with care plans; they do not have time to read them. Or that the care plans are too long to read and don't seem much to do with what is actually happening in the care situation.

There seem to be a number of practical issues that need to be addressed and some underlying key principles which need to be taken on board. The practical issues relate to communication and time management and the key principles are to do with the values and beliefs held by the care provider. We use the term 'care provider' here to mean the organisation providing the care. This might be a health or social care provider such as a primary care trust or borough council, a not-for-profit voluntary organisation, or a private family, or residential or nursing home.

COMMUNICATION

For a care plan to be implemented, the people giving the care and the person receiving it need to know what's in the care plan and, ideally, to have been involved in the process. The plan needs to communicate clearly what the person's needs are and the action the carer needs to take to meet them. All too often, written instructions such as 'needs assistance' are vague and non-specific. A well-written plan should be able to guide a relative stranger through the actions they need to take to support the person in an individualised way.

These actions can be communicated in writing very clearly if the SMART rules are applied. So, when documenting actions in the 'My carers will' column of the Enriched Care Plan you need to ensure that what you document is:

S   Specific

M   Meaningful

A   Agreed

R   Realistic

T   Time based

Specific means exact and precise. The phrase 'My carers will provide assistance to help me get dressed' is not specific and fails to communicate individualised interventions to the carer. A specific instruction would be explicit about the assistance needed and any carer working only with the vague instruction of giving assistance runs a high risk of getting off to a bad start.

As an example, the enriched profiling process for James has revealed that he does not like the idea of being given assistance to dress. Furthermore, he doesn't like to get dressed in the morning, he likes to stay in his pyjamas and will only consider changing his clothes if family are visiting, or if he is going out. He is happy to change into clean pyjamas at any time of the day or night if they need changing because he likes to stay feeling fresh and clean. This comes from a lifelong habit of liking to own many sets of good quality cotton pyjamas; of changing into his pyjamas as soon as he got home from work; and preferring to wear pyjamas in the house when relaxing. James' personality is such that he doesn't stick with set routines but he likes to be in control and to make his own choices. Cognitively, he operates comfortably in 'goal-directed' mode but needs verbal and visual prompts to start off a course of action, including changing his clothes.

This all needs to be communicated in his care plan. So, to be specific, you might start by thinking about short tailored instructions, such as:

My carers will:

- tell me when my family are visiting, or if I am going out and then ask me if I want to change my clothes for the day

- show me two clean shirts to choose from

- respect that I wish to wear good quality clean pyjamas during the day when I am relaxing and at night when I go to sleep

- prompt me to take off my old items when my pyjamas or clothes need changing

- place all the clothes I need to change into on my bed.

A **Meaningful** action is one that is important to the person. Being provided with 'assistance' is not meaningful to James whereas being helped to look smart and appropriate when his family visit him and being given a choice of shirt is.

The support to be provided also needs to be **Agreed**. James has agreed to his carers helping him with dressing, but only in keeping with *his* values which are to look smart when out and about or receiving visitors but to wear comfortable cotton pyjamas during the day when relaxing.

This instruction for James' carers is **Realistic** because it is likely to be achievable; a plan that, for example, instructed carers to dress James up in a shirt and tie every day would be unrealistic because James would resist this and refuse to co-operate.

Finally, the documentation within the Enriched Care Plan for supporting James needs to be **Time based**. There are two aspects to this, firstly when and how often the action needs to be done and secondly, when it will be reviewed. There is a third column on the far right hand side of the Enriched Care Plan for writing the review date if this is appropriate.

To complete James' plan for dressing following the SMART rules, a review date needs to be set, probably within 6–8 weeks would be appropriate – and you would write this in the far right hand column. More detail about how often and when the carer(s) need to help James needs to be added in to finalise the documentation:

My carers will:

- daily, after breakfast, remind me if my family are visiting, or if I am going out

- daily, after breakfast and whenever my pyjamas or clothes look dirty, ask me if I want to change them

- show me two clean shirts to choose from whenever you are helping me to change from my pyjamas into day wear

- at all times respect that I wish to wear clean good quality clean cotton pyjamas during the day when I am relaxing as well as at night when I go to sleep

- whenever I need and agree to a change of clothes or pyjamas, please prompt me to take off my old items and put on the new ones

- whenever helping me to change, leave the clean clothes I am to wear on my bed.

All documentation within the Enriched Care Plan should be written in clear plain English following the SMART rules so that they make sense to all who read them, including the person. The plan must also be communicated verbally in handovers and at case reviews.

TIME MANAGEMENT

A crucial factor for successful implementation of the Enriched Care Plan is time. Time for profiling, identifying needs, documenting needs, reviews and for regular face-to-face communication between all concerned needs to be ring fenced and costed in by the care provider. If this is not considered to be important, the care plan is unlikely to be effectively implemented and all the time taken to profile and document the person's needs will not give you the required outcome which is to deliver person-centred care.

KEY PRINCIPLES

Perhaps, to view effective communication and time management as important, the care provider (personal carers and their organisation) must truly value 'the person' at the centre of the enriched care planning process.

This brings us back to where we started in Chapter 1 where we used the VIPS Model to understand the principles of person-centred care. We need to look at these principles again now as we think about moving forward all the hard work you have done during the stages of profiling the person and identifying their needs towards a care plan that can be implemented and actually improve matters for the person who is living with dementia.

Using the VIPS Model for implementing and reviewing the Enriched Care Plan

V **V**aluing people applies not only to the person being cared for but also the people providing the care. This means that, when you write the Enriched Care Plan, you need to think about who is going to read it and who is going to implement it – these might not be the same people. It should be written in simple language, spelling out clearly what is expected of who and how often; it should be written in language that is respectful and non-judgemental. This means that *any* person reading it, especially the person for whom it has been written, will feel comfortable, supported, understood and respected as they read it.

I The Enriched Care Plan should be **I**ndividualised which means it will be different from everybody else's plan. The person's own name should be used throughout and their needs identified and documented in the context of their own profile of their unique life story, lifestyle and future wishes, personality, health, capacity for doing, cognitive ability and life at the moment.

P There may be several different **P**erspectives coming into the forefront during the process of enriched care profiling and planning but the plan itself should reflect the perspective of the person. This is why writing the Enriched Care Plan in the first person, as 'I', is recommended.

S **S**ocial living makes for an enriched life. For this reason, the enriched plan needs to focus just as much, if not more, on what the person needs to live their life as a social being as on concrete things like medication and physical care.

Reviewing the plan has been briefly mentioned already. This is crucial for two reasons. First as a way of checking that what is happening as a result of the Enriched Care Planning process is improving matters for the person. Second the Enriched Care Plan needs to be reviewed so that it is kept current and relevant.

There are no fixed rules for how often a review should be done. The single most important consideration is, in our opinion, whether or not the current plan is going well. We consider it good practice for all carers to keep an eye on this, to regularly observe how the person is doing and communicate with the person about how things are going. The carers who are in regular contact are usually in a good position to do this. In this way, the review process is kept alive as an ongoing and important process. More formal and regular reviews are also necessary. Some teams review routinely every six months or every year, while others only review if there is a problem or a change for the person. Probably a combination of both of these is a good idea.

SUMMARY

- How well care plans are implemented and reviewed will depend on the value and importance given to this process in your work setting.

- The practicalities of how communication is handled and how much time is allocated is the responsibility of the care provider.

- Documentation in the Enriched Care Plan should be SMART (Specific, Meaningful, Agreed, Realistic, Time based).

- The VIPS Model can be used as a set of principles to underpin the implementation and review of the enriched care planning process.

CONCLUSION

In writing this good practice guide, we have drawn from our own experiences but also, importantly, we have been inspired and informed by the work of our many colleagues in the world of dementia care. We are also fortunate to be able to use material from the immense body of current knowledge relating to the physical, psychological and social aspects of 'humanness'. This is highly relevant in helping us to understand dementia which is undeniably a human condition and therefore part of ordinary life.

Our work for the Bradford Dementia Group over the past few years has gifted us with the great privilege of learning from paid and family carers and professionals all of whom have helped to shape our vision for enriched care planning and motivated us to keep going with our writing.

Most importantly though, we must continue to listen to our fellow human beings who live with dementia if we are to succeed in working together to make person-centred care a reality:

> …this fact that we live in the present, with a depth of spirit and some tangled emotions, rather than cognition, means you can connect with us at a deep level…we live in the present reality, with no past and no future. We put all of our energy into *now*, not then or later. (Bryden 2005, p.99)

Useful Resources

Action for Advocacy
PO Box 31856
Lorrimore Square
London
SE17 3XR
Tel: 020 7820 7868
Fax: 020 7820 9947
Email: info@actionforadvocacy.org.uk
www.actionforadvocacy.org.uk

Age Concern
Age Concern England
Astral House
1268 London Road
London
SW16 4ER
Free helpline: 0800 00 99 66
www.ageconcern.org.uk

Age Exchange
The Reminiscence Centre
11 Blackheath Village
London
SE3 9LA
Tel: 020 8318 9105
Fax: 020 8318 0060
Email: administrator@age-exchange.org.uk
www.age-exchange.org.uk

Bladder & Bowel Foundation (formerly the Continence Foundation)
SATRA Innovation Park
Rockingham Road
Kettering
Northants
NN16 9JH
Nurse helpline for medical advice:
0845 345 0165

Counsellor helpline: 0870 770 3246
General enquiries: 01536 533255
Fax: 01536 533240
Email: info@bladderandbowelfoundation.org
www.bladderandbowelfoundation.org

Bradford Dementia Group
University of Bradford
School of Health Studies
University of Bradford
25 Trinity Road
Bradford
BD5 0BB, UK.
Tel: +44 01274 236367
Fax: +44 01274 236302
E mail: enquiries@bradford.ac.uk
www.bradford.ac.uk

British Dental Association
64 Wimpole Street
London
W1G8YS
Tel: 020 7935 0875
Fax: 020 7487 5232
Email: enquiries@bda.org
www.bda.org

British Dietetic Association
5th Floor, Charles House
148/9 Great Charles Street Queensway
Birmingham
B3 3HT
Tel: 0121 200 8080
Fax: 0121 200 8081
Email: info@bda.uk.com
www.bda.uk.com

British Medical Association (BMA)
BMA head office
BMA House
Tavistock Square
London
WC1H 9JP
Tel: 020 7387 4499
Fax: 020 7383 6400
Download information about accessing medical
records: http://www.bma.org.uk/ap.nsf/
Content/Access2007

Chartered Society of Physiotherapy
14 Bedford Row
London
WC1R 4ED
Tel: 020 7306 6666
www.csp.org.uk

College of Occupational Therapists
106-114 Borough High Street
Southwark
London
SE1 1LB
Tel: 020 7357 6480
www.cot.co.uk

College of Optometrists
42 Craven Street
London
WC2N 5NG
Tel: 020 7839 6000
Fax 020 7839 6800
Email: optometry@college-optometrists.org
www.college-optometrists.org

Department of Health (Medical Records)
The Department of Health
Richmond House
79 Whitehall
London
SW1A 2NS
Tel: 020 7210 4850
www.dh.gov.uk

Direct gov
Directgov is the website of the UK government
providing information and online services for
the public.
www.direct.gov.uk

**Federation of Ophthalmic and Dispensing
Opticians (FODO)**
199 Gloucester Terrace
London
W2 6LD
Tel: 020 7298 5151
Email: optics@fodo.com
www.fodo.com

JPA (Jackie Pool Associates) Limited
Sunnybanks
Victoria Road
Bishops Waltham
Southampton
SO32 1DJ
Tel: 01489 892933
Fax: 01489 890147
www.jackie-pool-associates.co.uk

**MIND (National Association for Mental
Health)**
PO Box 277
Manchester
M60 3XN
Tel: 0845 766 0163
Email: info@mind.org.uk
www.mind.org.uk

**The Office of the Public Guardian and the
Court of Protection**
Archway Tower
2 Junction Road
London
N19 5SZ
Tel: 0845 330 2900 - Phone lines are open
from 9am – 5pm
Fax: 020 7664 7705
www.publicguardian.gov.uk

**Personal Social Services Research Unit
(PSSRU)**
PSSRU at Kent
Cornwallis Building
George Allen Wing
University of Kent
Canterbury
Kent
CT2 7NF
Tel: 01227 827672
Fax: 01227 827038
Email: pssru@kent.ac.uk

PSSRU at the LSE

LSE Health and Social Care

London School of Economics and Political
Science

Houghton Street

London

WC2A 2AE

Tel: 020 7955 6238

Fax: 020 7955 6131

Email: pssru@lse.ac.uk

PSSRU at Manchester

University of Manchester

First Floor

Dover Street Building

Oxford Road

Manchester

M13 9PL

Phone: 44 (0) 161 275 5250

Fax: 44 (0) 161 275 5790

Email: pssru@man.ac.uk

www.pssru.ac.uk

Download Factsheet on
Pain from www.pssru.ac.uk/pdf/MCpdfs/Pain_
factsheet.pdf

Royal College of Nursing

20 Cavendish Square

London

W1G 0RN

Telephone: 020 7409 3333

www.rcn.org.uk

Royal College of Physicians

11 St Andrew's Place

Regent's Park

London

NW1 4LE

Tel: 020 7224 1539

Fax: 020 7487 5218

Email: infocentre@rcplondon.ac.uk

The Abbey Pain Scale is available to download
from the RCP website at
www.rcplondon.ac.uk/pubs/contents/ff4dbcd6-
ffb7-41ad-b2b8-61315fd75c6f.pdf

**Royal College of Speech and Language
Therapists**

2 White Hart Yard

London

SE1 1NX

Company registration number 518344

VAT number 795 811977

Tel: 020 7378 1200

Email: info@rcslt.org

www.rcslt.org

**Royal Pharmaceutical Society of Great
Britain**

1 Lambeth High Street

London

SE1 7JN

Tel: 020 7735 9141

Fax: 020 7735 7629

Email: enquiries@rpsgb.org

www.rpsgb.org.uk

The Royal College of Psychiatrists

National Headquarters

17 Belgrave Square

London

SW1X 8PG

Tel: 020 7235 2351

Fax: 020 7245 1231

E mail : rcpsych@rcpsych.ac.uk

www.rcpsych.ac.uk

The Society of Chiropodists and Podiatrists

Registered Office

1 Fellmonger's Path

Tower Bridge Road

London

SE1 3LY

Tel: 020 7234 8620

Fax: 0845 450 3721

www.feetforlife.org

✔

Life Story Profile for:

Completed by:

On:

Early Years
Memories of Family and Friends

My grandparents:

My parents:

My brothers and sisters:

Other people:

Memories of Schooling and Education

My talents and interests:

My friends and teachers:

My achievements and dreams:

Stories from my Early Years:

Middle Years

Memories of Family and Friends

Weddings, births and other special days:

Difficult times and sad days:

Memories of Things I Did

My work:

My hobbies and holidays:

Stories from my Middle Years:

After Retirement

Memories of Family and Friends

Weddings, births and other special days:

Difficult times and sad days:

Memories of Things I Enjoyed

Work, hobbies and travel:

Special places and special things:

Stories from After Retirement:

Now
Who and What I Think About

Proudest achievements:

Best day:

Regrets:

Happiest memories:

Recent Stories:

154

Lifestyle and Future Wishes Profile for:
Completed by: **On:**

Food and drinks that I like:

When and how I like to eat:

Clothes I like to wear:

My routines for daily living activities:

Work-like activities that I need to do routinely:

How I relax:

People, places or objects that I feel attached to:

What I do and what I need to help me feel close to them:

My spirituality:

Copyright © Hazel May, Paul Edwards and Dawn Brooker 2008

If I cannot communicate my wishes at any time in the future

Please take into account these lifestyle preferences:

I would be happy to accept the following additional treatments/support:

I would prefer not to accept the following additional treatments/support:

I want the following person/people to be consulted about my treatment/support at the time such decisions need to be made:

I have/have not made an Advance Directive or Living Will

The original document is held at:

Copies are held by:

I have/have not appointed someone as an 'attorney' to make decisions on my behalf.

My Property and Affairs Attorney is:

My Personal Welfare Attorney is:

My LPA has/has not been registered with the Office of the Public Guardian.

My original LPA documents are held by:

Copies are held by:

Personality Profile for:

Completed by:

On:

How I see myself – put an X where you think you sit on each line and then make comments

secure, confident _____ sensitive, nervous

Comments:

shy, withdrawn _____ outgoing, energetic

Comments:

cautious, conservative _____ inventive, curious

Comments:

competitive, outspoken _____ friendly, compassionate

Comments:

easy-going, carefree _____ efficient, organised

Comments:

Health Profile for:

Completed by: **On:**

My current health issues include:

These are the treatments I have:

These are the medications, substances and situations that cause me to have an allergic reaction:

My current weight is:

I am/am not happy with my weight

I do/do not smoke	**I do/do not drink alcohol**
Amount per day: Tobacco	**Alcohol**

Profile	Special needs	I would like a specialist assessment (tick if yes) →	
Eating			
Drinking			
Communicating			
Moving about			
Using the toilet			
Sleeping			

Profile

Profile	Date of last check up:	Special needs	I would like a specialist assessment (tick if yes) →
Eyes and vision			
Ears and hearing			
Teeth and gums			
Heart and lungs			
Feet			
Skin			
Women's*/men's* health issues * Delete as appropriate			

Pain:

Risks:

My Mental Health and Well-being

I do/do not feel depressed sometimes

I do/do not feel anxious sometimes

I do/do not experience other unpleasant feelings sometimes

More information that I want people to know about, including things people have said or done in the past to help me with these feelings:

I have/have not been given a diagnosis to explain my memory problems

Diagnosed on: .... (date)

by: .... (name)

My particular symptoms:

How I wish others to refer to this condition:

I would/would not like further specialised cognitive assessments

Further information about my physical or mental health that I would like other people to know about:

Capacity for Doing Profile for:
Completed by: On:

	I manage this well	Sometimes this is difficult	I'm not sure	Please ask my carer
Automatic actions				
I am able to:				
Turn my head				
Open my mouth				
Swallow				
Postural actions				
I am able to:				
Drink from a cup placed in my hand				
Pick up food with my fingers				
Use one implement to eat				
Manual actions				
I am able to:				
Reach out and grasp one eating implement				
Cut my food with one eating implement				
Separate or mash my food with one eating implement				
Goal-directed actions				
I am able to:				
Use **two** eating implements together to eat				
Use **two** implements together and cut my food with my knife				

My Comments:

Cognitive Ability Profile for:
Completed by: On:

	This happens to me sometimes	This doesn't happen to me	I'm not sure	Please ask my carer
Visual processing				
I see only part of what is in front of me				
I see things that other people don't see				
I find it hard to find the object I am looking for, even when it is right in front of me				
Everyday objects look strange or unrecognisable				
Body management and awareness				
It is difficult for me to start getting dressed or undressed on my own without someone to prompt me				
It is difficult for me to choose my clothes from my wardrobe/dresser spontaneously				
It is difficult for me to co-ordinate my arms and body parts during washing or dressing				
It is difficult for me to know exactly where my arms or legs are during washing or dressing				
Memory				
I have difficulty remembering what I have seen				
I have difficulty remembering what has been said to me				
I have difficulty recognising				
• faces of people I know				
• familiar objects				
• familiar surroundings				

	This happens to me sometimes	This doesn't happen to me	I'm not sure	Please ask my carer
I have difficulty remembering the layout of where I am				
I have difficulty remembering where I have put things				
Communication				
I have difficulty starting off talking				
I have difficulty stopping talking				
It is difficult for me to reply when people talk to me				
I lose track of what I am talking about				
I can't think of the word I want				
It is difficult for me to understand what is being said to me				
Planning, judging and controlling				
I find it difficult to focus on what I want to do				
It is difficult for me to plan ahead				
I find it difficult to learn anything new				
It is difficult for me to start off on a course of action				
It is difficult for me to stop what I am doing				
I have trouble controlling my emotions				
I have trouble controlling my impulses				

These are the comments I would like to make:

Life at the Moment Profile for:
Completed by:

On:

My level of satisfaction about my life here

These are my feelings, about living my life here:

I want you to ask somebody else (Name):
to speak for me and write what they say here:

My Psychological Needs

Generally in my day-to-day living here	Not met at all	Minimally and/or infrequently met	Moderately or sometimes met	Met to a considerable extent and/or often	Met fully and/or always	Comments
My need for comfort is						
My need for occupation is						
My need for attachment is						
My need for identity is						
My need for inclusion is						

Enriched Profile and Care Plan for:

People who have helped me:

Place:

Date:

Brief Profile Sheet for:

I need	My carers will	We will review this on

Brief Profile Sheet for:

Important Issues Relating to my Life Story:

Important Issues Relating to my Lifestyle and Future Wishes:

My Personality:

Key Health and Risk Issues:

My Capacity for Doing:
My predominant way of engaging with the world at the current time is:

Automatic	Postural	Manual	Goal Directed

My Cognitive Ability:
I need help with:

Visual Processing	Body Management	Memory	Communicating
Initiation	Planning	Judging	Controlling

My Life at the Moment:

Significant well-/ill-being issues for immediate attention:

My satisfaction with the care I get here:

My carer or significant other's satisfaction with the care I get here:

My psychological needs:

Key Information Sheet

Name that I wish to be called by:

My date of birth .... **Age** ....

People that I may wish to contact:

Name	Address/Contact details	Relationship to me	Additional information

Important information that I want people involved in my care to know about:

The Enriched Care Plan

I need	My carers will	We will review this on

References

Abbey, J. (2007) 'The assessment of pain in older people.' *Concise Guidance to Good Practice.* London: Royal College of Physicians.

Allan, K. (2001) *Communication and Consultation: Exploring Ways for Staff to Involve People with Dementia in Developing Services.* London and Bristol: Policy Press and Joseph Rowntree Foundation.

Allen, C.K., Earhart, C.A. and Blue, T. (1992) *Occupational Therapy Treatment Goals for the Physically and Cognitively Disabled.* Rockville USA: The American Occupational Therapy Association.

Alzheimer's Society (2008) *Dementia out of the Shadows.* London: Alzheimer's Society.

Ballard, C., Fossey, J., Chithramohan, R., Howard, R., *et al.* (2001) 'Quality of care in private sector and NHS facilities for people with dementia: cross sectional survey.' *British Medical Journal 323,* 426–427.

Barnett, E. (2000) *Including the Person with Dementia in Designing and Delivering Care 'I Need to be Me!'* London and Philadelphia: Jessica Kingsley Publishers.

Brod, M., Stewart, A.L., Sands, L. and Walton, P. (1999) 'Conceptualization and measurement of quality of life in dementia: the Dementia Quality of Life Instrument (DQOL).' *The Gerontologist 39,* 1, 25–35.

Brooker, D. (2004) 'What is person-centred care in dementia?' *Reviews in Clinical Gerontology 13,* 3, 215–222.

Brooker, D. (2006) *Person-Centred Dementia Care: Making Services Better.* London: Jessica Kingsley Publishers.

Brooker, D., Woolley, R. and Lee, D. (2007) 'Enriching opportunities for people living with dementia in nursing homes: an evaluation of a multi-level activity-based model of care.' *Aging and Mental Health 11,* 4, 361–370.

Browne, C. J. and Shlosberg, E. (2006) 'Attachment theory, ageing and dementia: a review of the literature.' *Aging and Mental Health 10,* 2, 134-142.

Bruce, E. (1998) 'How can we measure spiritual well being?' *Journal of Dementia Care 6,* 3, 16–17.

Bryden, C. (2005) *Dancing with Dementia: My Story of Living Positively with Dementia.* London: Jessica Kingsley Publishers.

Continence Foundation (2008) Continence Symptoms and Treatments. Available at www.continence-foundation.org.uk/symptoms-and-treatments/bowel.php#6, accessed on 16 February 2009.

Disability Foundation (2006) www.tdf.org.uk/therapies/chiropody.htm, accessed on 16 February 2009.

Edvardsson, D., Winblad, B. and Sandman, P.O. (2008) 'Person-centred care of people with severe Alzheimer's disease: current status and ways forward.' *The Lancet Neurology 7,* 4, 362–367.

Fiske, J., Frenkel, H., Griffiths, J. and Jones, V. (2006) 'Guidelines for the development of local standards of oral health care for people with dementia.' *Gerodontology 23,* 1, available at www.gerodontology.com

Harris, P. B. (ed.) (2002) *The Person with Alzheimer's Disease: Pathways to Understanding the Experience.* London and Baltimore: Johns Hopkins University Press.

Heath, H. (1999) 'Intimacy and sexuality.' In H. M. B. Heath and I. Schofield (eds) *Healthy Ageing: Nursing Older People.* London: Mosby, pp.341-366.

Kitwood, T. (1997) *Dementia Reconsidered: The Person Comes First (Reconsidering Ageing)*. Buckingham, PA: Open University Press.

Keady, J. (1996) 'The experience of dementia: a review of the literature and implications for nursing practice.' *Journal of Clinical Nursing 5*, 275-288.

Miesen, B. (1993) 'Alzheimer's disease, the phenomenon of parent fixation and Bowlby's attachment theory.' *International Journal of Geriatric Psychiatry 8*, 147-153.

Miesen, B. (1997) 'Care giving in demetia; the challenge of attachment'. In Jones, G. *Caregiving in Dementia*, vol 2. London, New York: Routledge.

McCrae, R.R. and Costa, P.T. Jr (2003) *Personality in Adulthood: A Five-Factor Theory Perspective* (2nd edn). New York: Guildford Press.

Mozley, C.G., Hukley, P., Sutcliffe, C. and Bayley, H. (1999) '"Not knowing where I am doesn't mean I don't know what I like!" Cognitive impairment and quality of life responses in elderly people.' *International Journal of Geriatric Psychiatry 14*, 9, 776–783.

Nagaratnam, N. and Gayagay, G. (2002) 'Hypersexuality in nursing home facilities: a descriptive study.' *Archives in Gerontology and Geriatrics 35*, 3, 195–203.

Passmore, P. (2005) 'Behavioural and psychological symptoms in Alzheimer's disease.' *Journal of Quality Research in Dementia 1*, 12.

Perrin, T., May, H. and Anderson, L. (2008) *Wellbeing in Dementia: An Occupational Approach for Therapists and Carers*. Edinburgh: Churchill Livingstone.

Personal Social Services Research Unit (2005) Pain in Dementia Factsheet www.pssru.ac.uk/pdf/MCpdfs/Pain_factsheet.pdf

Phares, E.J. (1991) *Introduction to Psychology* (3rd edition). New York: Harper Collins Publishers.

Pool, J. (2007) *The Pool Activity Level (PAL) Instrument for Occupational Profiling: A Practical Resource for Carers of People with Cognitive Impairment (Bradford Dementia Group Good Practice Guides)*. London: Jessica Kingsley Publishers.

Powell, J. (2000) *Care to Communicate: Helping the Older Person with Dementia*. London: Hawker Publications.

Royal College of Psychiatrists (2008) www.rcpsych.ac.uk/mentalhealthinformation/ mentalhealthproblems/sleepproblems/sleepingwell.aspx, accessed on 16 February 2009.

Sabat, S. (2001) *The Experience of Alzheimer's Disease: Life Through a Tangled Veil*. Oxford: Blackwell.

Smeeth, L, Fletcher, A.E., Stirling, S., Nunes, M., *et al.* (2001) 'Randomised comparison of three methods of administering a screening questionnaire to elderly people: findings from the MRC trial of the assessment and management of older people in the community.' *British Medical Journal 323*, 1403.

Society of Chiropodists and Podiatrists (2008) 'Feet for Life' foot health info web page, www.feetforlife.org/foot_health/common_probs.html/, accessed on 22 June 2009.

Surr, C. (2006) 'Preservation of the self in people with dementia living in residential care: a socio-biographical approach.' *Social Science and Medicine 62*, 7, 1720–1730.

Wallace, M. (1992) 'Management of sexual relationships among elderly residents of long-term care facilities.' *Geriatric Nursing 13*, 6, 308–311.

Young, A. and Dinan, S. (1994) 'ABC of Sports Medicine: fitness for older people.' *British Medical Journal 309*, 331–334.

Index